The Low

FODMAP

DIET

COOKBOOK

A simple guide to gut-friendly recipes to beat blot and heal your IBS symptoms and other digestive disorder

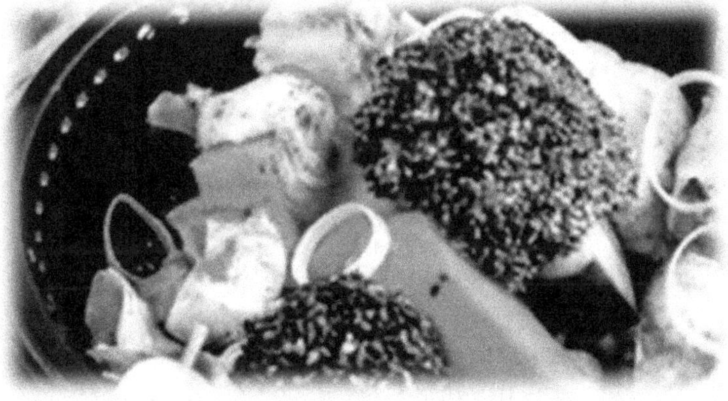

Dr. Grace Hester

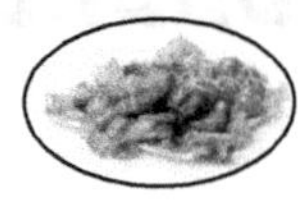 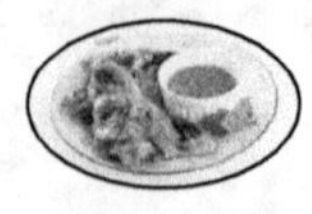 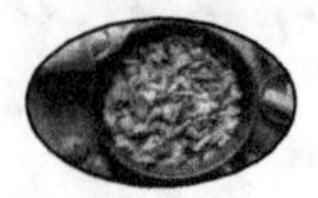

Copyright Page

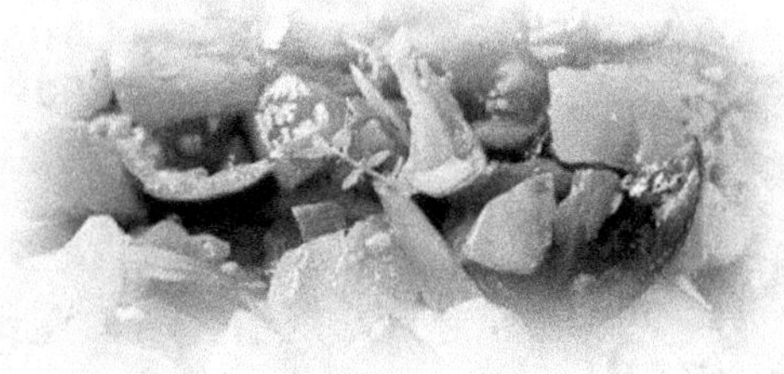

DR. GRACE HESTER

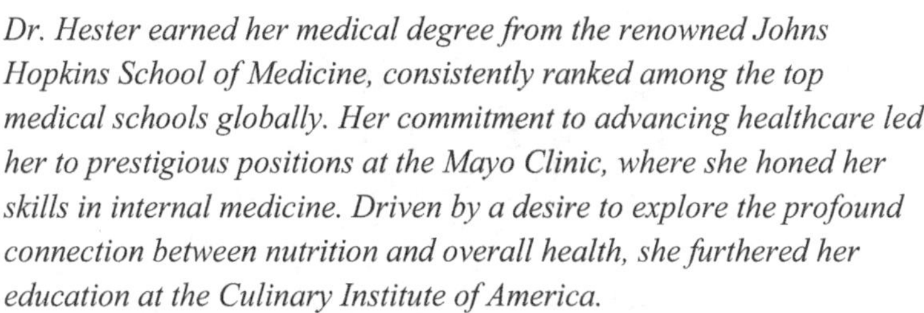

Dr. Grace Hester stands at the intersection of health, passion, and culinary excellence. A distinguished medical professional and accomplished nutritionist, she seamlessly weaves together her expertise to create a holistic approach to well-being.

Dr. Hester earned her medical degree from the renowned Johns Hopkins School of Medicine, consistently ranked among the top medical schools globally. Her commitment to advancing healthcare led her to prestigious positions at the Mayo Clinic, where she honed her skills in internal medicine. Driven by a desire to explore the profound connection between nutrition and overall health, she furthered her education at the Culinary Institute of America.

– With a deep understanding of both medicine and nutrition, Dr. Hester embarked on a mission to inspire others to embrace a healthier lifestyle. Her culinary journey– led to the creation of a series of cookbooks that blend the art of cooking with the science of nutrition. Each recipe is a testament to her commitment to flavor, nourishment, and well-being.

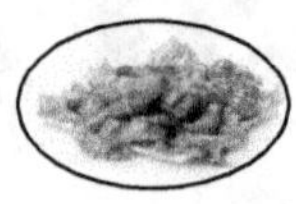
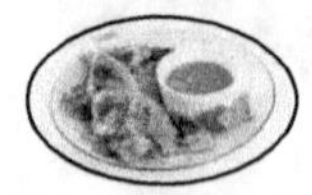
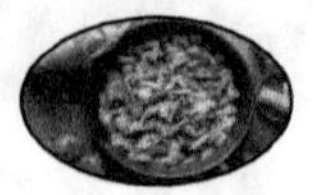

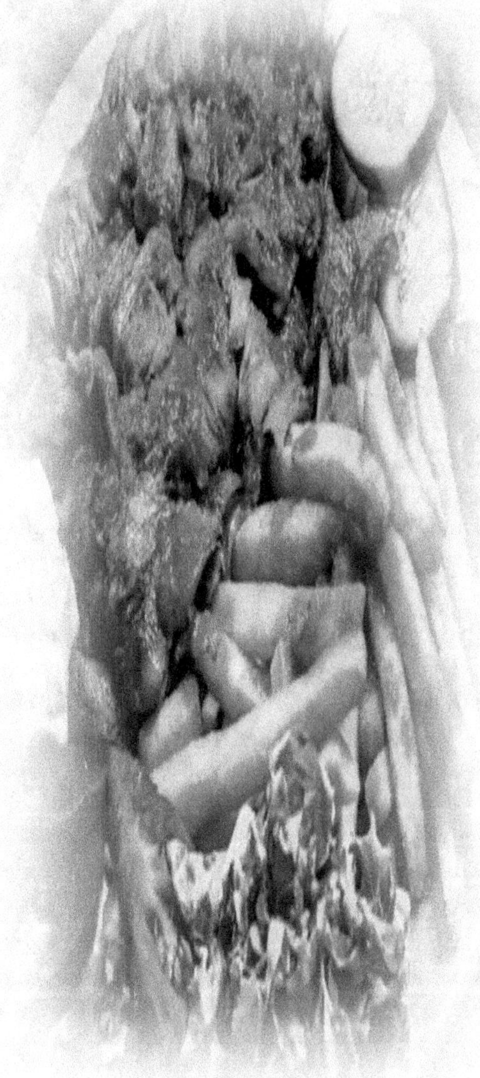

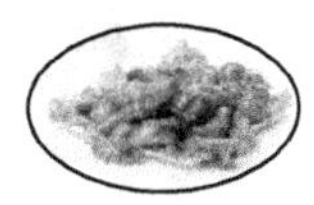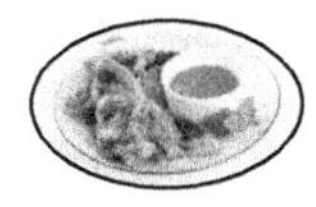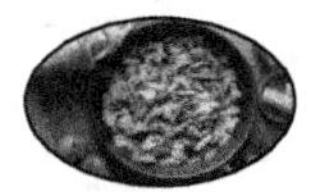

TABLE OF CONTENT

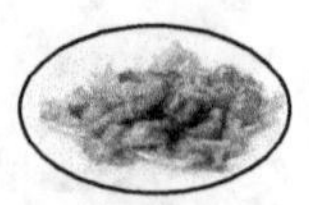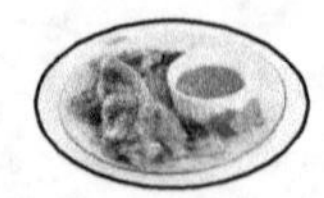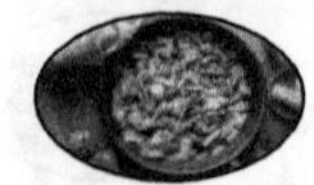

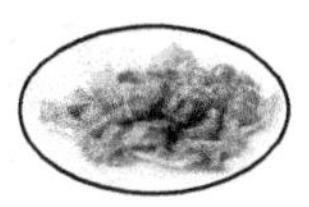
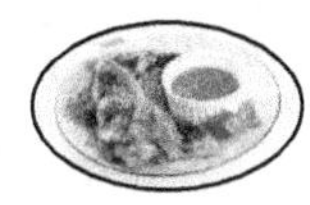
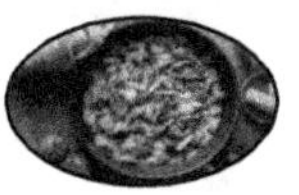

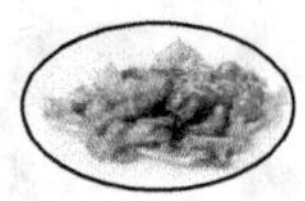 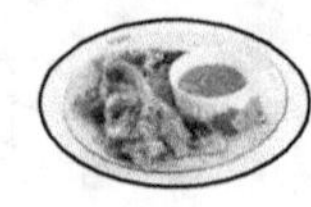 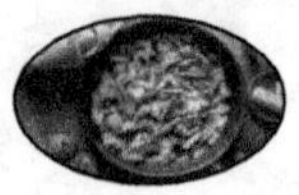

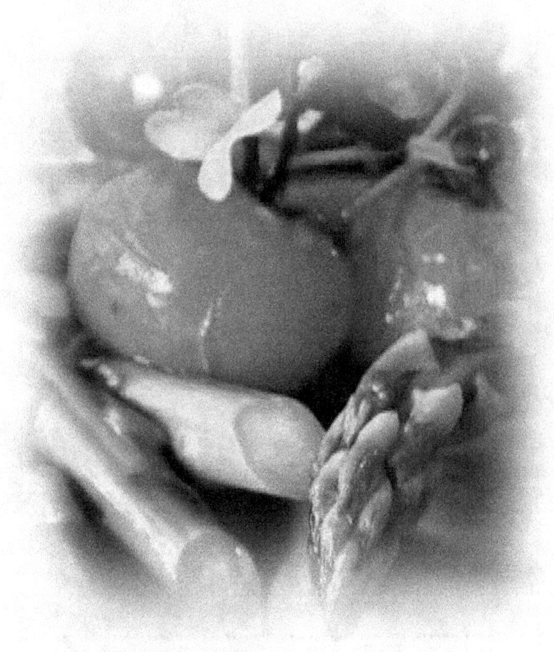

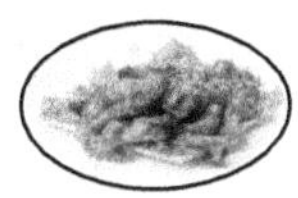 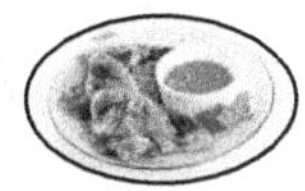 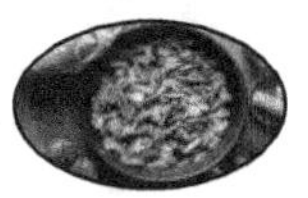

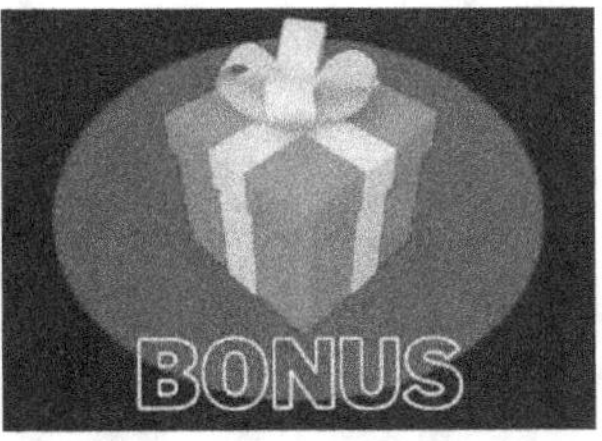

SCAN THE QR CODE TO GET YOUR FREE HOME MADE GREEN SMOOTHIE RECIPE BOOK

Your 20 days meal planner is attached at the end of the book. Enjoy!

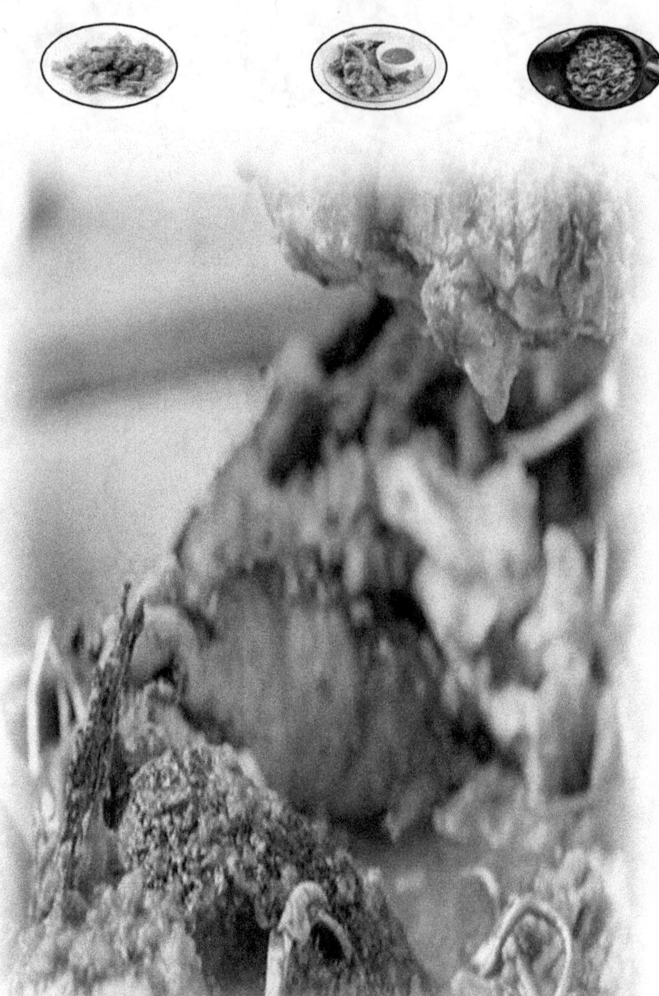

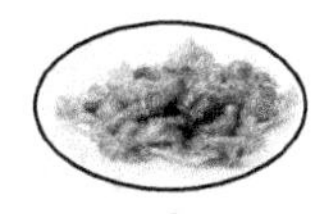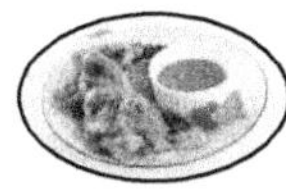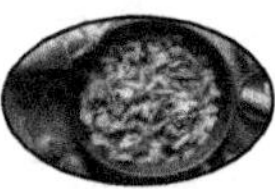

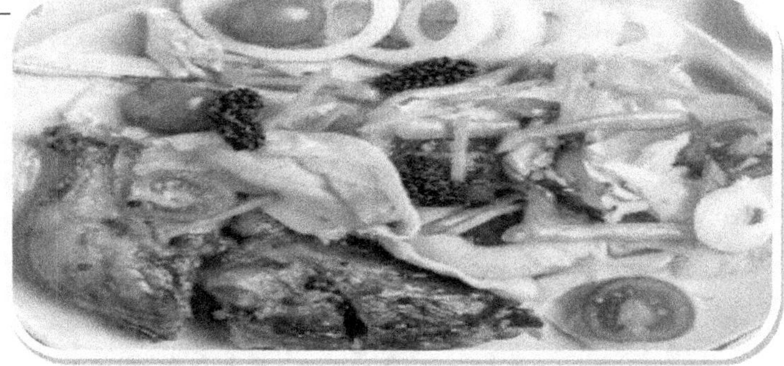

FORWARD

Are you looking to manage your digestive health and alleviate persistent digestive symptoms? The solution you've been searching for may lie in the Low FODMAP Diet. This book serves as a comprehensive guide, grounded in scientific support, to help you embark on this dietary approach and gain control over digestive disorders like irritable bowel syndrome (IBS).

Discover more about FODMAPs and their impact on digestive health in "The Low FODMAP Diet for Beginners." Uncover insights on ensuring you receive all necessary nutrients while adhering to the diet, along with practical guidance on menu planning, grocery shopping, and dining out.

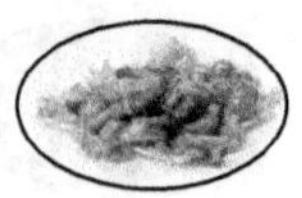 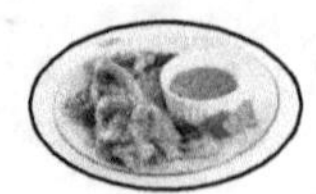 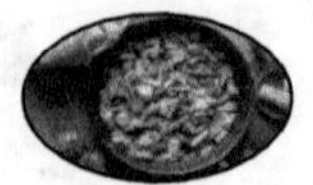

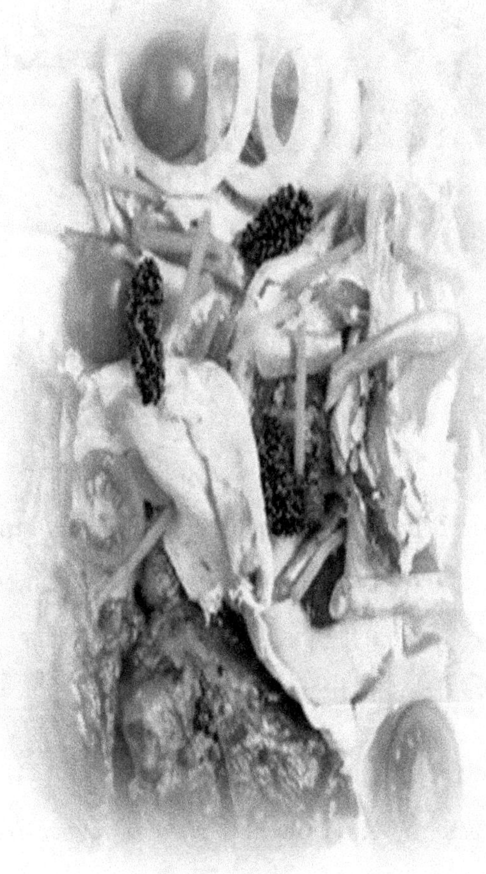

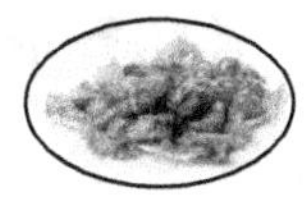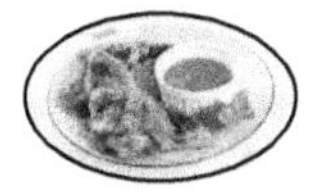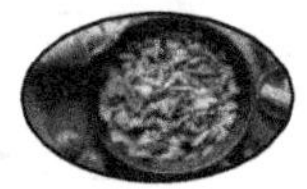

INTRODUCTION

Since my teenage years, I've witnessed my mother's struggle with Irritable Bowel Syndrome (IBS) and Small Intestinal Bacterial Overgrowth (SIBO). Constantly plagued by bloating and abdominal pain, she experimented with various diets and therapies without success until she stumbled upon the Low FODMAP Diet.

Initially skeptical due to perceived limitations, my mother's health began to improve after a few weeks on the Low FODMAP Diet. Witnessing this transformation, I delved into researching the diet, realizing it was not as restrictive as believed. Collaborating with my mother, we devised a personalized Low FODMAP Diet strategy, and as a dietitian, I began sharing my knowledge with others.

Motivated by my personal and my mother's success, I decided to compile this book, "The Low FODMAP Diet for Beginners," a comprehensive guide to understanding and implementing the Low FODMAP Diet to improve your quality of life.

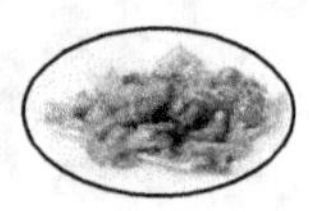 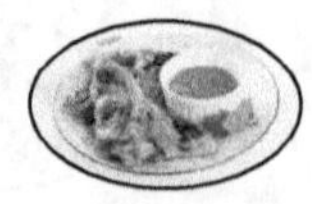 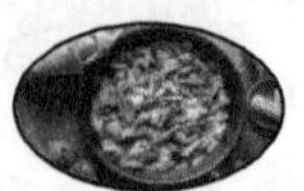

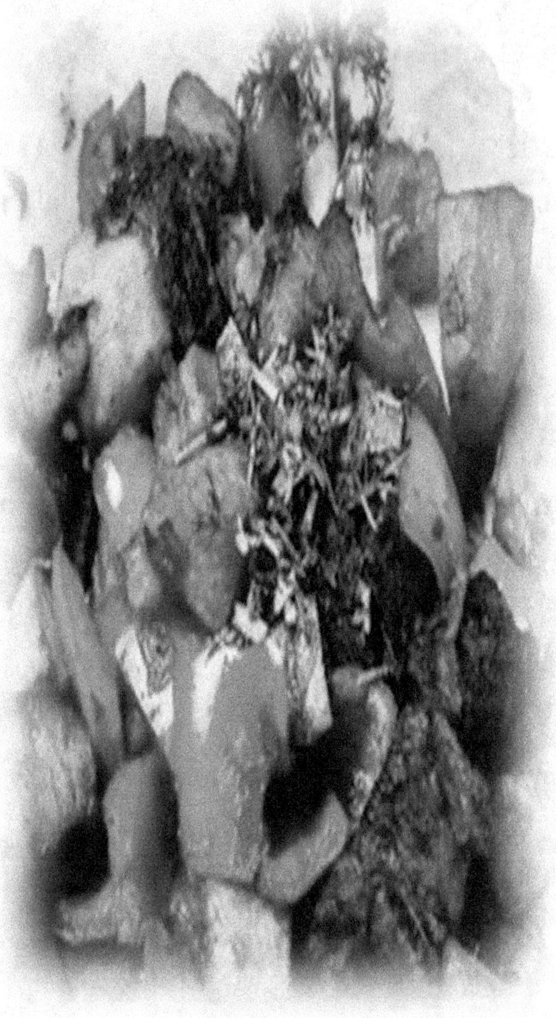

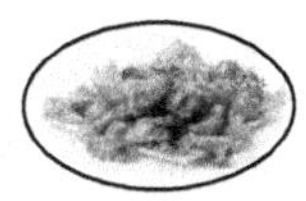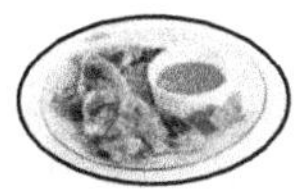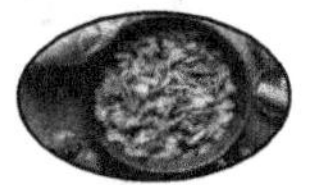

CHAPTER ONE

THE LOW FODMAP DIET: WHAT IS IT?

The Low FODMAP Diet is a dietary strategy designed to alleviate the symptoms of IBS by restricting the intake of specific carbohydrates known as FODMAPs. These carbohydrates, including fermentable oligosaccharides, disaccharides, monosaccharides, and polyols, are challenging to digest and can ferment in the gut, leading to digestive pain.

The diet comprises two phases: initially removing FODMAPs for 6 to 8 weeks, followed by gradually reintroducing small amounts to identify tolerated and non-tolerated FODMAPs. While effective for many, individual variations exist, and collaboration with a healthcare professional is essential to tailor the approach. Maintaining a balanced diet and ensuring adequate nutrient intake are crucial considerations.

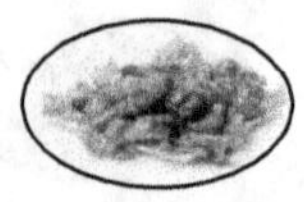 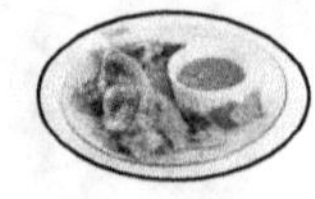 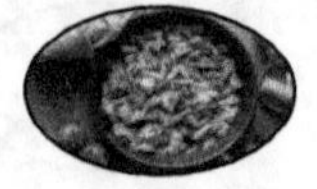

BENEFITS OF A LOW FODMAP DIET

The Low FODMAP Diet is specifically designed to manage IBS symptoms and other digestive disorders, offering several benefits. By reducing FODMAP intake, individuals can alleviate symptoms such as bloating, stomach pain, constipation, and diarrhea, significantly improving their overall quality of life.

This diet is not exclusive to IBS and extends its benefits to other digestive diseases like Crohn's disease and ulcerative colitis. Additionally, it supports weight management by reducing overall calorie consumption, fostering a diet rich in whole foods and minimizing processed food intake.–

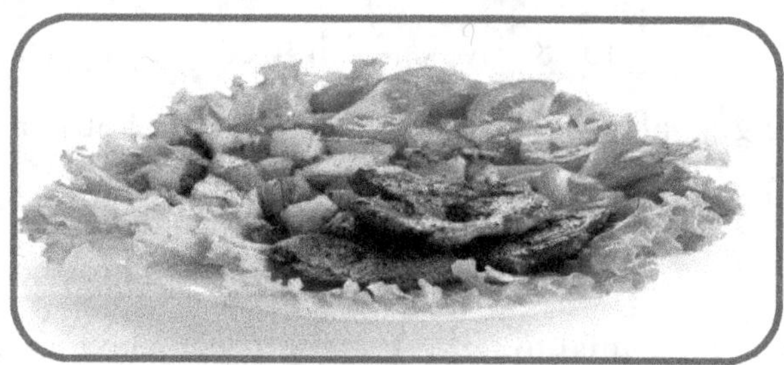

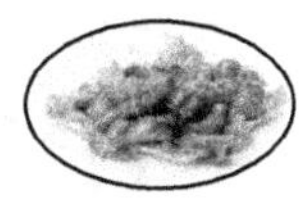 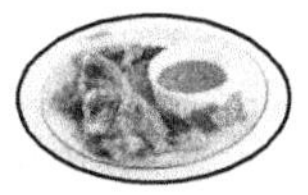 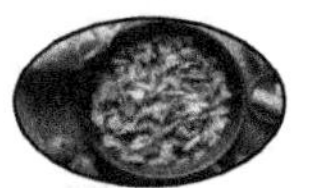

CHAPTER TWO

FOODS TO STEER CLEAR OF ON A LOW FODMAP DIET

The Low FODMAP Diet restricts various FODMAP-rich foods to alleviate symptoms associated with digestive diseases. Foods like wheat, onions, garlic, apples, pears, and specific vegetables and legumes should be avoided due to their difficulty in small intestine absorption, leading to abdominal discomfort.

While some foods are prohibited, the diet allows for alternatives like lactose-free milk, certain fruits and vegetables, and gluten-free grains. Notable exclusions encompass barley, rye, beans, cashews, and pistachios.

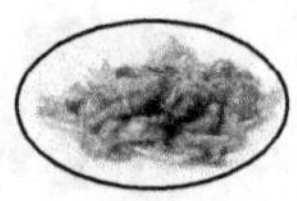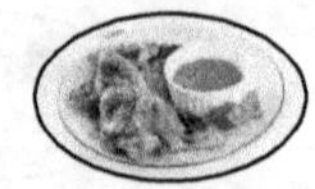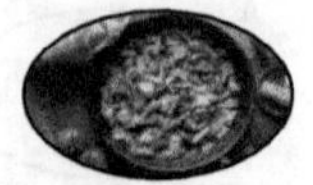

CHAPTER THREE

BREAKFAST, SMOOTHIES, AND DRINKS RECIPES FOR LOW FODMAP

Berry Smoothie (FODMAP-friendly)

Ingredients:

- 1/4 cup frozen blueberries and raspberries

- 1/2 cup almond milk

- 1/2 cup plain yogurt

- 1 tablespoon honey

- 1/4 teaspoon ground cinnamon

Instructions:

1. Add all ingredients to a blender and process until smooth.

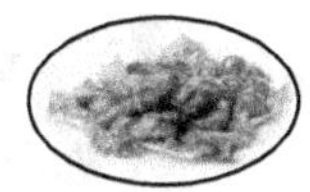 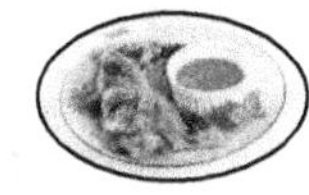 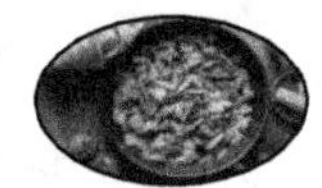

2. Serve immediately.

Green Smoothie (Low FODMAP)

Ingredients:

- 1/2 banana

- 1/4 cup pineapple

- 1 cup spinach

- 1/2 cup almond milk

- 1/2 cup plain yogurt

- 1 teaspoon honey

- 1/4 teaspoon ginger root

Instructions:

1. Combine all elements in a blender and blend until smooth.

2. Serve immediately.

—

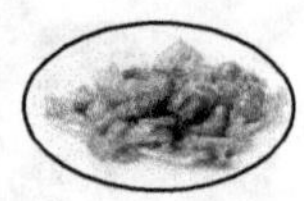 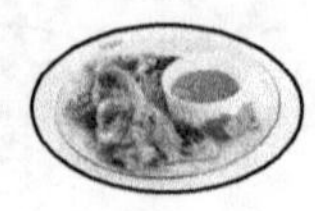 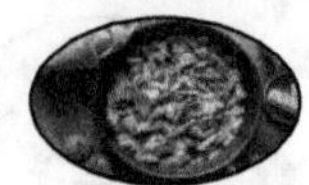

Healthy Banana Oatmeal

Ingredients:

- 1 1/2 cups rolled oats and mashed banana

- 1 cup almond milk

- 1 teaspoon cinnamon

- 1 tablespoon honey

Instructions:

1. Combine oats, mashed banana, almond milk, and cinnamon in a small saucepan.

2. Heat, stirring regularly, over medium heat until thick and creamy.

3. Turn off the heat and add honey.

4. Serve hot.

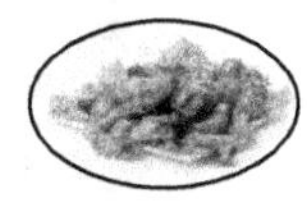 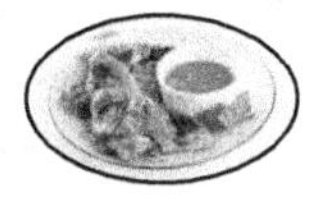 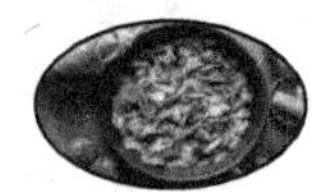

Ingredients:

- 1/4 cup chia seeds

- 1 cup almond milk

- 1/4 teaspoon ground cinnamon

- 1/2 teaspoon honey

- 1/2 teaspoon vanilla extract

Instructions:

1. Combine chia seeds, almond milk, cinnamon, honey, and vanilla in a medium bowl.

2. Stir to combine.

3. Refrigerate overnight or for at least two hours.

4. Serve cold.

—

Chia Pudding (Low FODMAP)

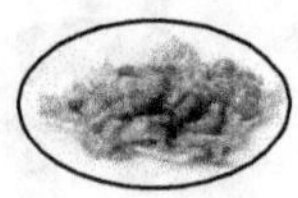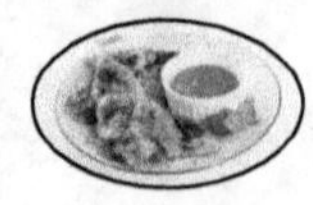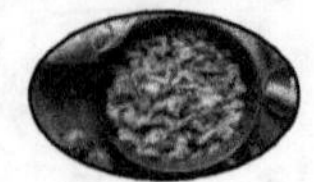

Ingredients:

- 1/2 cup all-purpose flour

- 1/2 teaspoon baking powder

- 1/4 teaspoon ground cinnamon

- 1/4 cup almond milk

- 1/2 shredded apple

- 1/4 teaspoon honey

Instructions:

1. Combine flour, baking powder, and cinnamon in a medium bowl.

2. In another bowl, combine almond milk, grated apple, and honey.

3. Add both liquid and dry ingredients and mix.

4. Cook spoonfuls of batter on a nonstick pan until golden brown.

5. Drizzle with honey and serve.

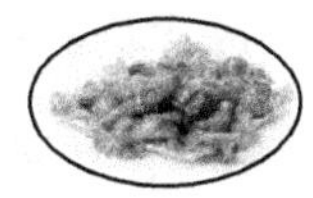 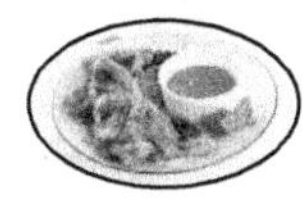 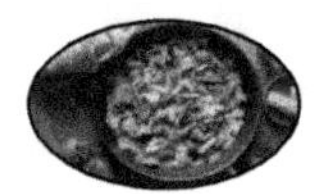

Avocado Toast (FODMAP-Friendly)

Ingredients:

- 1 slice gluten-free bread

- 1/2 mashed avocado

- 1/4 teaspoon garlic-infused olive oil

- 1/4 teaspoon sea salt

Instructions:

1. Toast the bread until golden brown.

2. Mash avocado in a bowl, add garlic-infused olive oil and sea salt.

3. Top toast with avocado mixture.

4. Serve immediately.

—

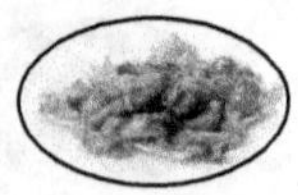 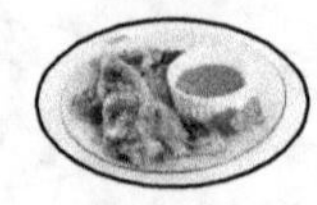 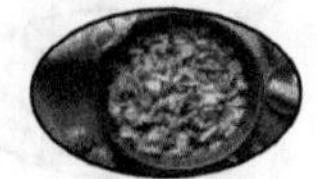

Ingredients:

- 1/4 cup each diced tomatoes, bell peppers, and onions

- 1/2 cup shredded cheese

- 6 eggs

- 1 clove garlic, infused olive oil

- 1/4 teaspoon sea salt

Instructions:

1. Preheat the oven to 350 degrees.

2. Grease a muffin tin.

3. Combine tomatoes, bell pepper, onion, cheese, eggs, garlic-infused olive oil, and sea salt.

4. Fill each muffin cup 3/4 full.

5. Bake until eggs are set, about 15 to 20 minutes.

6. Serve hot.

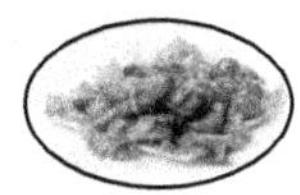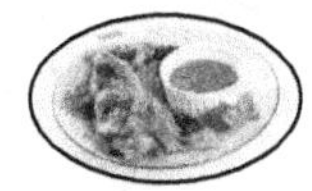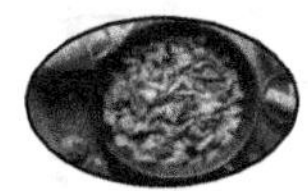

CHAPTER FOUR

SEAFOODS AND FISH FODMAP RECIPES

Salmon with Asparagus and Lemon

Preparation Time: 15 minutes

Cooking Time: 10 minutes

Ingredients:

- 4-6 ounces fresh salmon

- 2 tablespoons olive oil

- 1/2 teaspoon garlic-infused olive oil

- 2 tablespoons lemon juice

- One quarter teaspoon each of both salt and likewise black pepper–

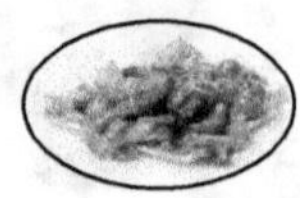 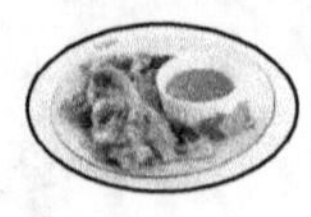 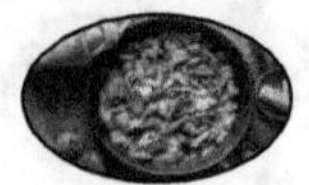

- 2 cups trimmed asparagus spears

- 1 lemon, thinly sliced

Instructions:

1. Preheat the oven to 370-375°F.

2. Place salmon on a baking pan.

3. Drizzle salmon with garlic-infused olive oil and regular olive oil.

4. Sprinkle with salt and pepper, then drizzle lemon juice over it.

5. Arrange asparagus spears around the salmon and top with lemon slices.

6. Bake for 10 minutes or until salmon is done.

7. Serve salmon with lemon slices and asparagus. Enjoy!

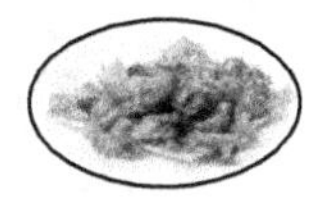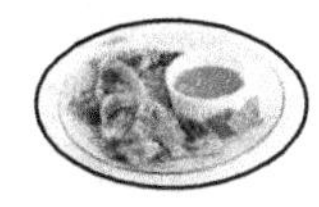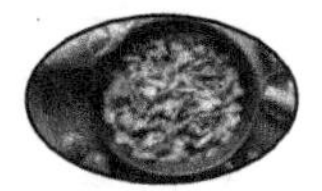

Preparation Time: 10 minutes

Cooking Time: 15 minutes

Ingredients:

- 4-6 ounces fresh halibut

- 2 tablespoons olive oil

- 1 teaspoon garlic-infused olive oil

- 1 teaspoon seasoned salt

- 1/4 teaspoon each of salt and black pepper

- 2 cups halved cherry tomatoes

Instructions:

1. Preheat the oven to 380-400°F.

2. Place halibut on a baking pan.

3. Drizzle halibut with olive oil and garlic-infused olive oil.

4. Season with salt, pepper, and Italian seasoning.

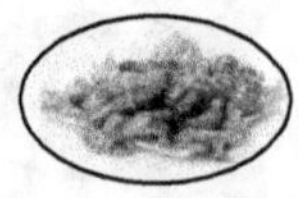 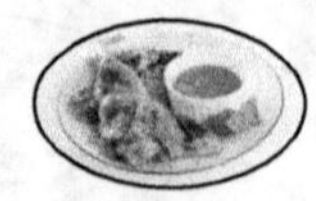 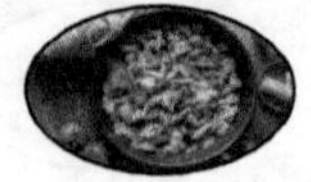

5. Surround the halibut with tomatoes.

6. Bake for 15 minutes or until thoroughly done.

7. Serve halibut with roasted tomatoes. Enjoy!

Roasted Potatoes and Tilapia

Preparation Time: 10 minutes

Cooking Time: 20 minutes

Ingredients:

- 4-6 ounces fresh tilapia

- 2 tablespoons olive oil

- 1 teaspoon garlic-infused olive oil

- 1 teaspoon seasoned salt

- One quarter teaspoon each of both salt and likewise black pepper

- 2 cups diced potatoes

–

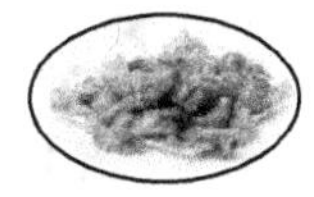 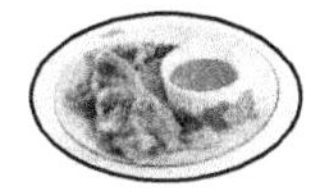 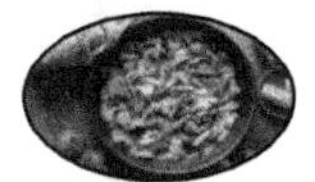

Instructions:

1. Preheat the oven to 375°F.

2. Place tilapia on a baking sheet.

3. Drizzle tilapia with olive oil and garlic-infused olive oil.

4. Season with salt, pepper, and Italian seasoning.

5. Surround the fish with potatoes.

6. Bake for 20 minutes or until thoroughly done.

7. Serve roasted potatoes with the tilapia. Enjoy!

Roasted Carrots and Shrimp

Cooking Time: 15 minutes

Ingredients:

- 1 teaspoon garlic

- 2 tablespoons olive oil

- half pound fresh shrimp, ensure it is peeled and also deveined

- 1 teaspoon seasoned salt

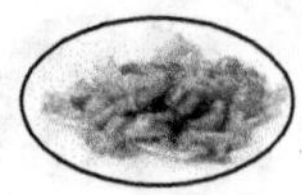 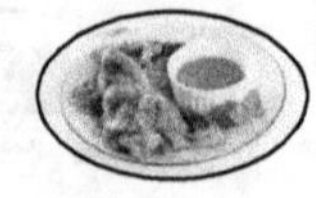 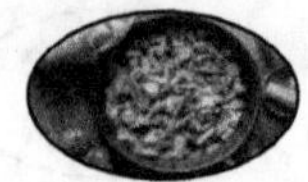

- 2 cups peeled and chopped carrots

- One quarter teaspoon each of both salt and likewise black pepper

Instructions:

1. Preheat the oven to 380-400°F.

2. Place shrimp on a baking pan.

3. Drizzle shrimp with garlic-infused olive oil and regular olive oil.

4. Season with salt, pepper, and Italian seasoning.

5. Surround the shrimp with carrots.

6. Bake for 14-16 minutes or when fully cooked.

7. Serve roasted carrots alongside the shrimp. Enjoy!

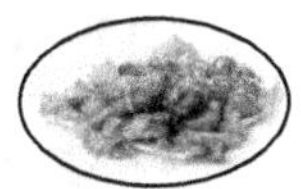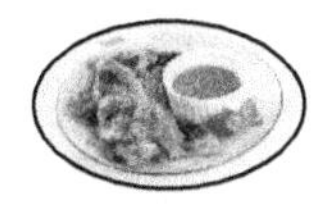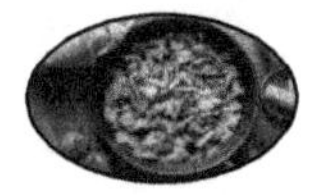

Scallops with Roasted Zucchini

Preparation Time: 10 minutes

Cooking Time: 10 minutes

Ingredients:

- 1 teaspoon garlic

- 2 tablespoons olive oil

- 1/2 pound fresh scallops

- 1 teaspoon seasoned salt

- One quarter teaspoon each of both salt and likewise black pepper

- 2 cups chopped zucchini

Instructions:

1. Preheat the oven to 380-400°F.

2. Place scallops on a baking sheet.

3. Drizzle scallops with regular olive oil and garlic-infused olive oil.

4. Season with salt, pepper, and Italian seasoning.

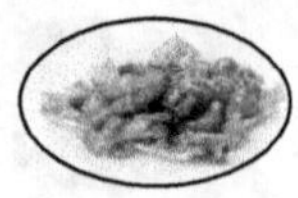 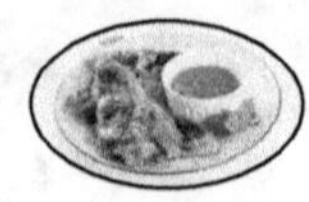 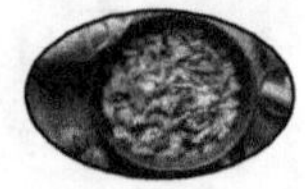

5. Arrange zucchini slices around the scallops.

6. Bake for 10 minutes or until fully cooked.

7. Combine roasted zucchini with the scallops. Enjoy!

Crab Cakes with Arugula Salad

Preparation Time: 15 minutes

Cooking Time: 10 minutes

Ingredients:

- 1 tablespoon garlic

- 2 tablespoons olive oil

- 1/2 pound fresh crab flesh

- 2 tablespoons gluten-free breadcrumbs

- 1/2 teaspoon salt

- 1/4 teaspoon black pepper

- 2 cups fresh arugula

- 1/4 cup lemon juice

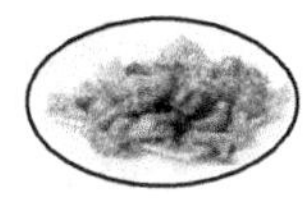 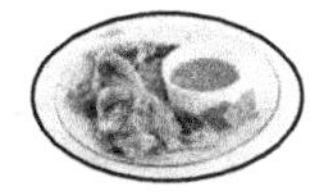 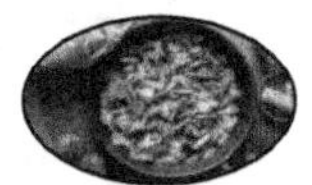

Instructions:

1. Combine breadcrumbs, olive oil, garlic-infused olive oil, salt, and crab meat in a big bowl.

2. Form patties from the mixture.

3. Cook crab cakes in a preheated skillet over medium heat until golden brown, about 5 minutes per side.

4. In a large bowl, combine arugula and lemon juice.

5. Place crab cakes on top of the arugula salad on serving plates. Enjoy!

Mussels in Garlic-Flavored Broth

Preparation Time: 10 minutes

Cooking Time: 15 minutes

Ingredients:

- 2 pounds fresh mussels

- 2 tablespoons olive oil

- 1/2 cup garlic-infused olive oil

- 1/2 glass of white wine

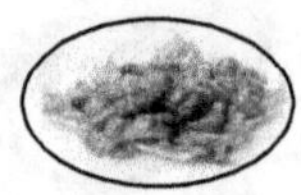 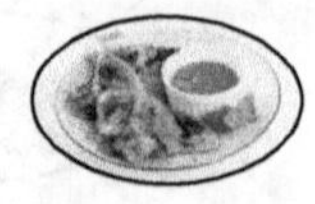 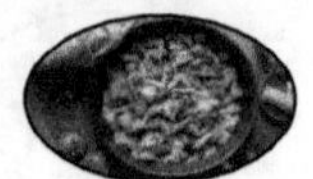

- 1 teaspoon seasoned salt

- One quarter teaspoon each of both salt and likewise black pepper

- Italian seasoning

Instructions:

1. Add olive oil to a big saucepan over medium heat.

2. Boil garlic-infused olive oil for one minute.

3. Add white wine, salt, pepper, Italian seasoning, and mussels.

4. Cook mussels covered for 10 to 15 minutes or until fully cooked.

5. Pour the garlic-flavored liquid over the mussels. Enjoy!

—

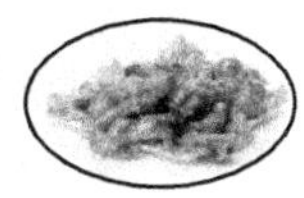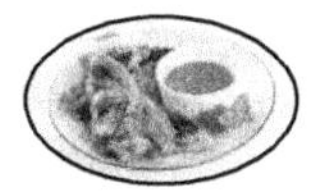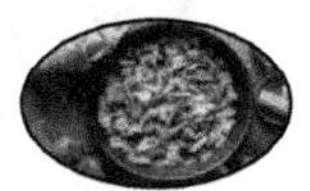

CHAPTER FIVE

MEAT LOW FODMAP RECIPES

Stir-Fried Chicken and Veggies

Instructions: Marinate chicken breasts in a low-FODMAP marinade like olive oil, garlic-infused oil, and oregano. Stir-fry chicken with prepared vegetables (carrots, bell peppers, mushrooms, and zucchini) and serve over cooked quinoa.

Baked Chicken Thighs with Potatoes and Spinach

Instructions: Marinate chicken thighs in low-FODMAP items like rosemary, ginger, and garlic-infused olive oil. Bake with potatoes, spinach, and other chosen veggies.

Herb and Lemon Roast Chicken

Instructions: Season a whole chicken with salt, pepper, and fresh herbs like thyme, parsley, and oregano. Serve with quinoa and roasted vegetables.–

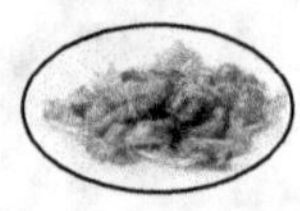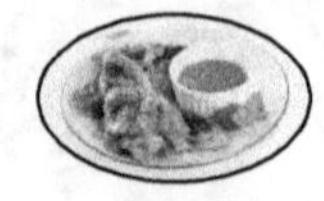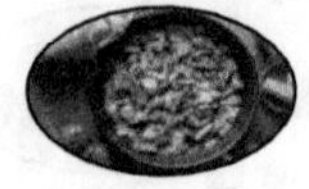

Grilled Chicken on Skewers with Squash and Zucchini

Instructions: Soak wooden skewers, then thread chicken, squash, and zucchini. Grill in a low-FODMAP marinade (olive oil, garlic-infused oil, and oregano) until thoroughly cooked.

Herbed Chicken with Rice and Broccoli

Instructions: Marinate chicken breasts in a low-FODMAP marinade (olive oil, garlic-infused oil, oregano). Serve over cooked brown rice and steamed broccoli after baking.

Honey Mustard Chicken

Instructions: Marinate chicken in honey, mustard, and garlic-infused oil before baking. Include steamed vegetables and quinoa.

Chicken and Eggplant Curry

Instructions: Prepare a low-FODMAP marinade (olive oil, garlic-infused oil, curry powder) for chicken breasts. Cook with preferred vegetables (eggplant, bell peppers). It can be Serve with brown rice or maybe a nice cooked quinoa.–

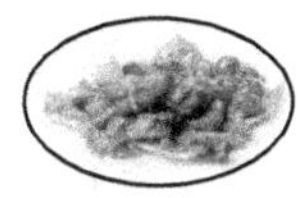 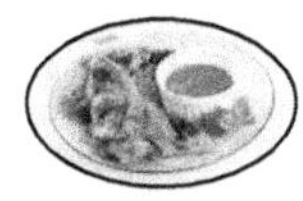 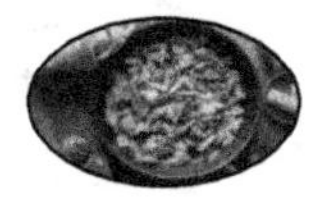

Roasted Chicken with Butternut Squash and Kale

Instructions: Prepare a marinade (olive oil, garlic-infused oil, oregano) for chicken breasts. Cook with kale and butternut squash. Serve with brown rice or cooked quinoa.

Chicken & Broccoli Quiche

Instructions: Prepare a low-FODMAP short-crust pastry. Fill with cooked chicken, broccoli, and additional vegetables. Serve hot or cold.

Chicken and Sweet Potato Casserole

Instructions: Prepare a low-FODMAP marinade (olive oil, garlic-infused oil, oregano) for chicken breasts. Add cooked sweet potatoes and other chosen vegetables. Bake thoroughly, then serve with a side salad.

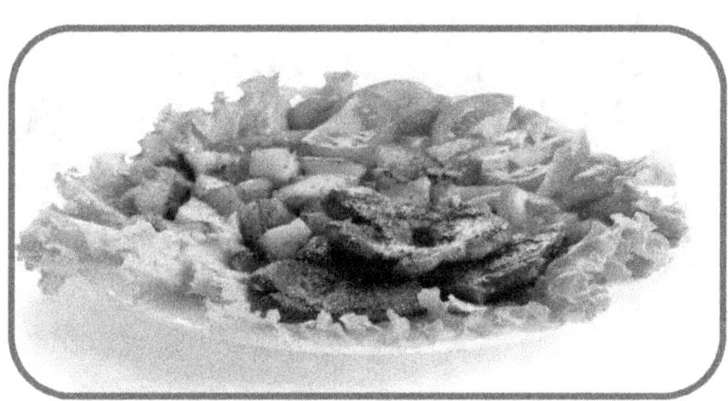

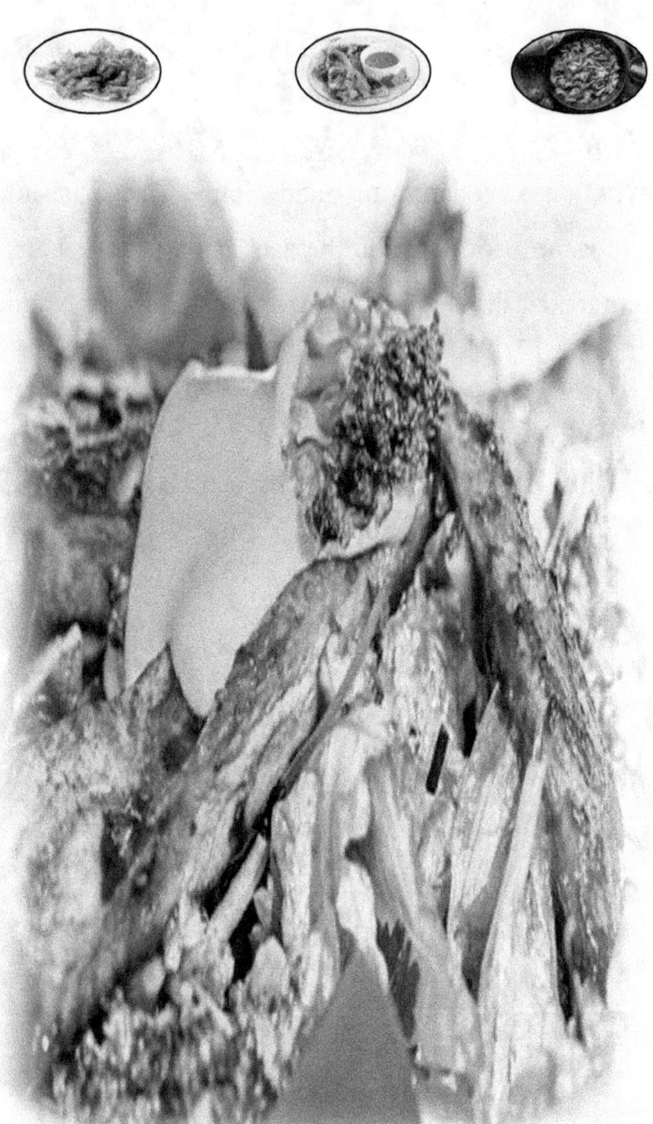

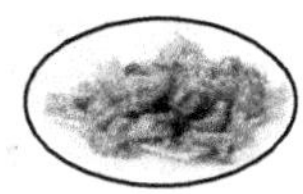 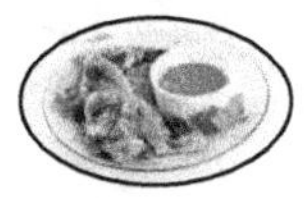 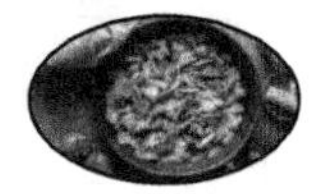

CHAPTER SIX

VEGETARIAN MAINS LOW FODMAP RECIPES

Quinoa Bowl with Roasted Veggies

Ingredients:

- 2 cups cooked quinoa

- 1 cup asparagus, chopped

- 1 cup bell peppers, sliced

- 1 cup zucchini, sliced

- 1 cup eggplant, diced

- 2 tablespoons olive oil

- Salt and pepper to taste

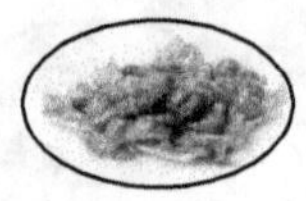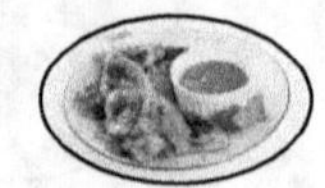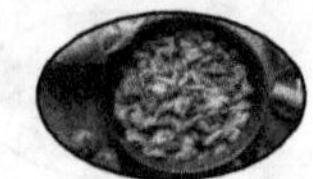

Instructions:

1. Preheat the oven to 350°F.

2. Combine asparagus, bell peppers, zucchini, and eggplant in a bowl.

3. Drizzle with olive oil, sprinkle with salt and pepper, and toss to coat.

4. Spread the veggies on a baking sheet and roast for 20 minutes.

5. Serve over cooked quinoa. Enjoy!

Creamy Polenta with Garlic-Infused Kale

Ingredients:

- 1 cup polenta

- 3 cups water

- 1 cup kale, chopped

- 2 tablespoons garlic-infused olive oil

- Salt and pepper to taste

- 1/2 cup non-dairy milk

Instructions:

1. Cook polenta according to package instructions using water.

2. In a separate pan, sauté kale in garlic-infused olive oil until wilted.

3. Season kale with salt and pepper.

4. Mix cooked polenta with non-dairy milk until creamy.

5. Serve polenta topped with garlic-infused kale. Enjoy!

Baked Eggplant with Vegan Cheese

Ingredients:

- 1 large eggplant, sliced

- 2 tablespoons olive oil

- Vegan cheese

- Marinara sauce

- Salt and pepper to taste

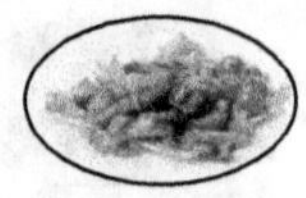 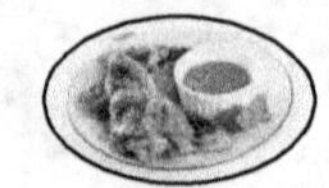 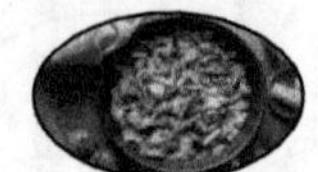

Instructions:

1. Preheat the oven to 375°F.

2. Coat eggplant slices with olive oil, salt, and pepper.

3. Bake for 25 -30 minutes or until well cooked.

4. Add a layer of vegan cheese on each slice and bake until melted.

5. Top with marinara sauce before serving. Enjoy!

Baked Sweet Potato Falafel

Ingredients:

- 1 cup cooked sweet potatoes, mashed

- 1 cup cooked chickpeas

- 1/2 cup flour (gluten-free)

- 1 teaspoon garlic

- 1 teaspoon cumin

- Tahini sauce

—

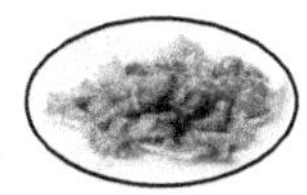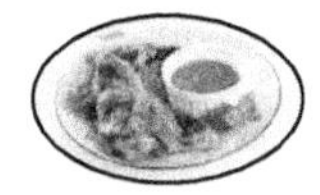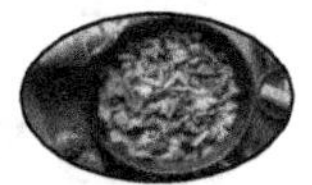

Instructions:

1. In a food processor, combine sweet potatoes, chickpeas, flour, garlic, and cumin.

2. Form small patties and place on a baking sheet.

3. Bake for 20 minutes at 350°F.

4. Serve with tahini sauce. Enjoy!

Zucchini Noodle Pasta with Pistachio Pesto

Ingredients:

- Zucchini noodles

- 1 cup fresh basil

- 1/4 cup pine nuts

- Vegan parmesan cheese

- 2 tablespoons olive oil

Instructions:

1. Spiralize zucchini into noodles.

2. In a blender, combine basil, pine nuts, vegan parmesan, and olive oil.

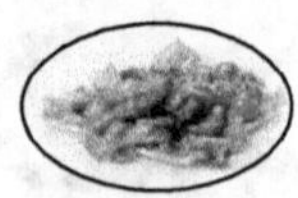 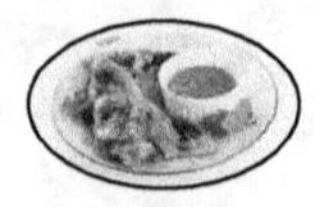 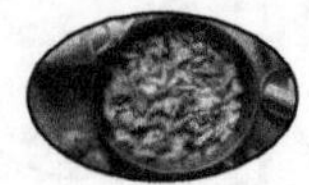

3. Toss zucchini noodles with pesto.

4. Garnish with additional pine nuts and vegan parmesan. Enjoy!

Lentil Tacos

Ingredients:

- 1 cup cooked lentils

- Salsa

- Cumin and chili powder to taste

- Taco shells

- Tomatoes, lettuce, avocado, vegan cheese for toppings

Instructions:

1. Season cooked lentils with salsa, cumin, and chili powder.

2. Fill taco shells with lentils.–

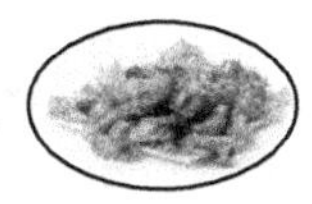 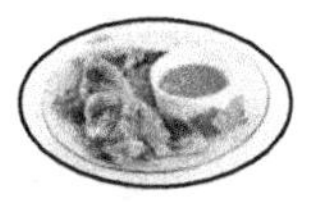 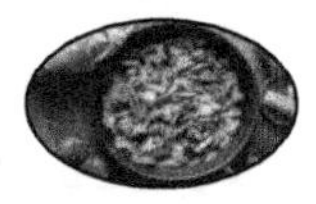

3. Top with tomatoes, lettuce, avocado, and vegan cheese. Enjoy!

Mushroom Risotto

Ingredients:

- Cooked risotto

- Mushrooms, sautéed in olive oil

- Fresh herbs

- Vegan parmesan cheese

Instructions:

1. Add sautéed mushrooms to cooked risotto.

2. Stir in fresh herbs and vegan parmesan cheese. Enjoy!

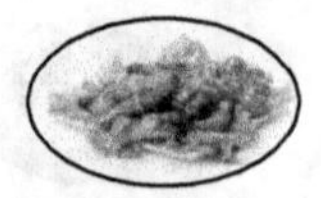 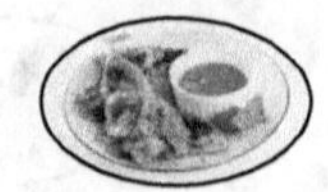 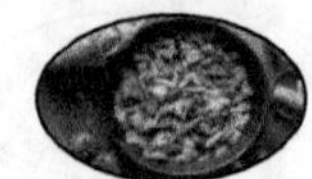

Quinoa Burgers

Ingredients:

- 1 cup cooked quinoa

- 1 cup mashed black beans

- 1/4 cup sliced onion

- Minced garlic to taste

- Seasonings

- Burger buns

Instructions:

1. Combine quinoa, mashed black beans, onion, garlic, and seasonings.

2. Form into patties and bake for 20 minutes at 350°F.

3. Serve on burger buns. Enjoy!

—

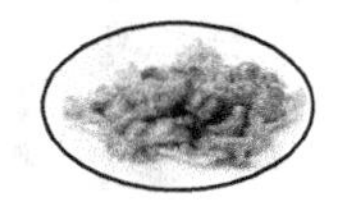 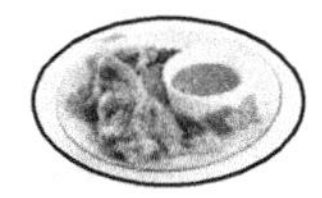 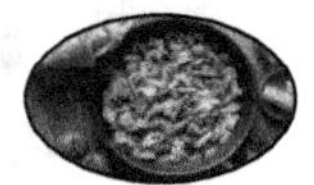

Ingredients:

- Portobello mushrooms, sliced

- Bell peppers, sliced

- Vegan cheese

- Salsa

- Guacamole

- Lettuce

Instructions:

1. Sauté Portobello mushrooms and bell peppers in oil.

2. Serve on a bed of lettuce with vegan cheese, salsa, and guacamole. Enjoy!

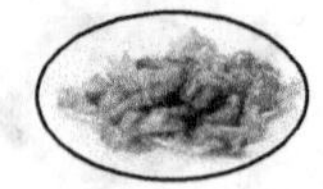 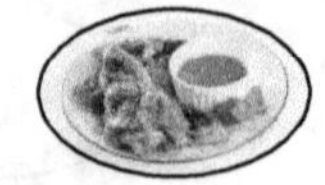 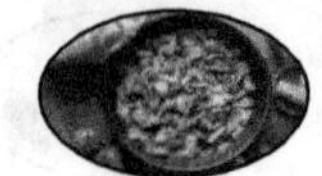

Eggplant Rollatini

Ingredients:

- Thinly sliced eggplant

- Tofu-ricotta cheese mixture

- Vegan cheese

- Herbs

Instructions:

1. Top eggplant slices with tofu-ricotta, vegan cheese, and herbs.

2. Roll up and bake for 20 minutes at 375°F. Enjoy!

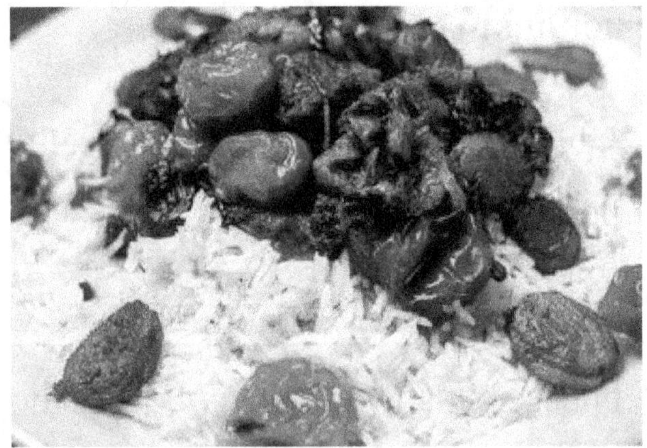

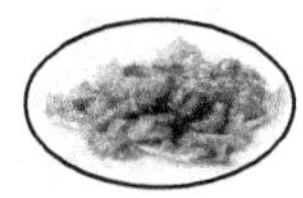 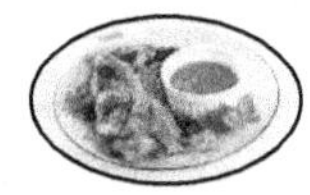 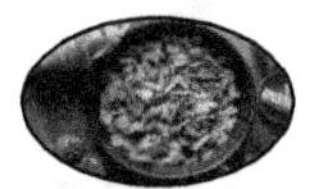

CHAPTER SEVEN

UNIQUE 2 WEEKS MEAL PLAN

DAY 1

- **Breakfast:** Banana-Berry Smoothie

- **Lunch:** Low-FODMAP Salad

- **Dinner:** Roasted Tomatoes and Salmon

DAY 2

- **Breakfast:** Low-FODMAP Overnight Oats

- **Lunch:** Lentil Soup

- **Dinner:** Low-FODMAP Pizza

DAY 3

- **Breakfast:** Low-FODMAP Granola

- **Lunch:** 10-Minute Prep Low-FODMAP Burrito Bowl–

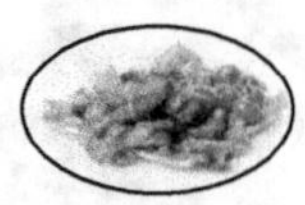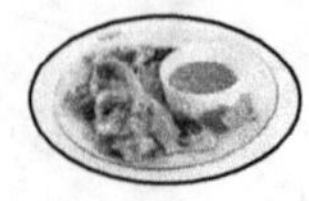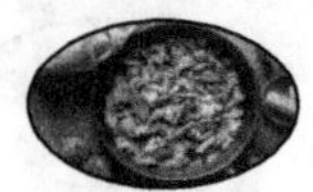

- **Dinner:** Low-FODMAP Chicken Stir-Fry–

DAY 4

- **Breakfast:** Low-FODMAP French Toast

- **Lunch:** Low-FODMAP Grilled Cheese

- **Dinner:** Low-FODMAP Veggie Wrap

DAY 5

- **Breakfast:** Low-FODMAP Yogurt Parfait

- **Lunch:** Low-FODMAP Avocado Toast

- **Dinner:** Low-FODMAP Roasted Vegetables

DAY 6

- **Breakfast:** Low-FODMAP Omelette

- **Lunch:** Low-FODMAP Soup

- **Dinner:** Low-FODMAP Sautéed Shrimp

DAY 7

- **Breakfast:** Low-FODMAP Granola Bar

- **Lunch:** Low-FODMAP Sandwich

- **Dinner:** Low-FODMAP Pizza–

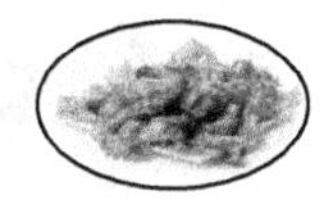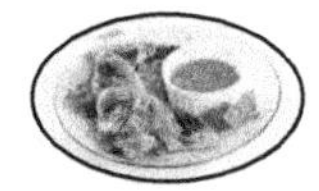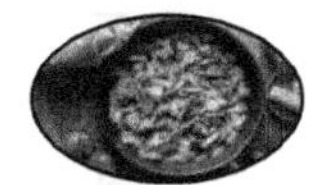

DAY 8

- **Breakfast:** Low-FODMAP Fruit Salad

- **Lunch:** Dinner in a Bowl of Quinoa

- **Dinner:** Low-FODMAP Stir-Fry

DAY 9

- **Breakfast:** Low-FODMAP Oatmeal

- **Lunch:** Low-FODMAP Rice Bowl

- **Dinner:** Low-FODMAP Chicken and Vegetables

DAY 10

- **Breakfast:** Low-FODMAP Smoothie

- **Lunch:** Low-FODMAP Burrito

- **Dinner:** Low-FODMAP Fish Tacos

DAY 11

- **Breakfast:** Low-FODMAP Pancakes

- **Lunch:** Low-FODMAP Sandwich

- **Dinner:** Low-FODMAP Ramen

DAY 12

- **Breakfast:** Low-FODMAP Muffins

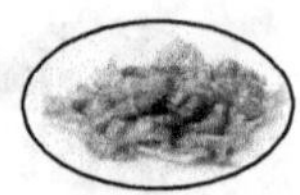 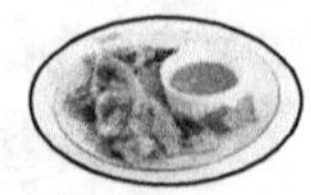 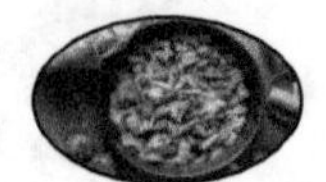

- **Lunch:** Low-FODMAP Salad

- **Dinner:** Low-FODMAP Curry

DAY 13

- **Breakfast:** Low-FODMAP Wraps

- **Lunch:** Low-FODMAP Granola

- **Dinner:** Low-FODMAP Pizza

DAY 14

- **Breakfast:** Low-FODMAP Soup

- **Lunch:** Low-FODMAP Yogurt Parfait

- **Dinner:** Low-FODMAP Pasta

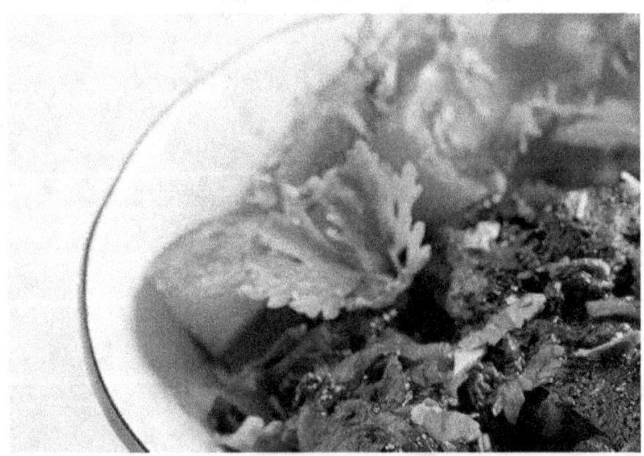

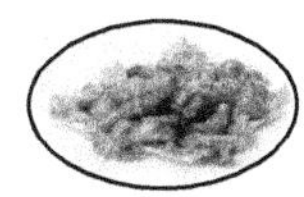 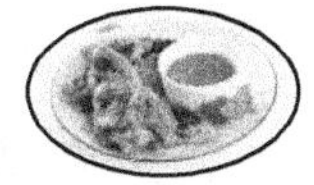 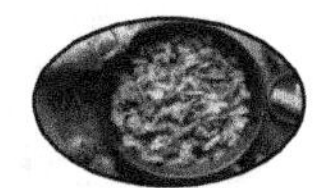

CHAPTER EIGHT

ADVICE FOR SIMPLIFYING THE LOW FODMAP DIET

1. **Make a Plan:**

    - Create a grocery list and meal plan before shopping.

2. **Use Your Imagination:**

    - Experiment with various ingredients and flavors.

3. **Low FODMAP Pantry:**

    - Stock up on low-FODMAP essentials like gluten-free grains, flours, beans, lentils, and quinoa.

4. **Learn to Read Labels:**

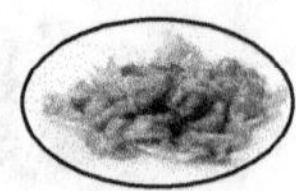 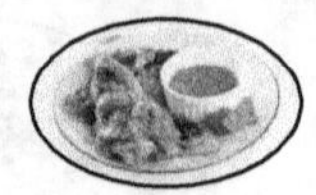 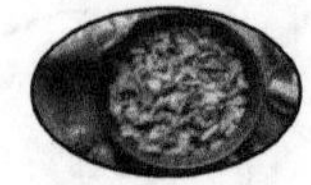

- Understand which foods are low in FODMAPs by reading food labels.

5. **Cook in Bulk:**

   - Prepare larger batches of food to have ready-made meals.

6. **Use Low FODMAP Recipes:**

   - Explore low-FODMAP recipes online.

7. **Seek Support:**

   - Join support groups or consult with a licensed dietitian.

8. **Monitor Your Progress:**

   - Keep a food log, planner or journal to track symptoms and identify those trigger foods.

—

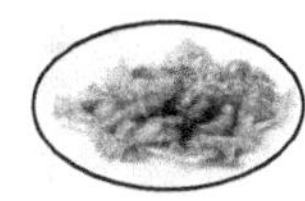 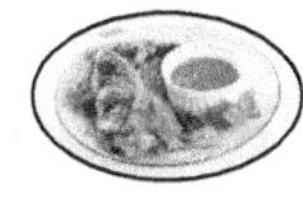 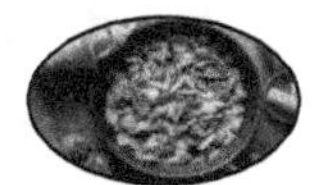

- **Email:** marionwrightbooks@gmail.com

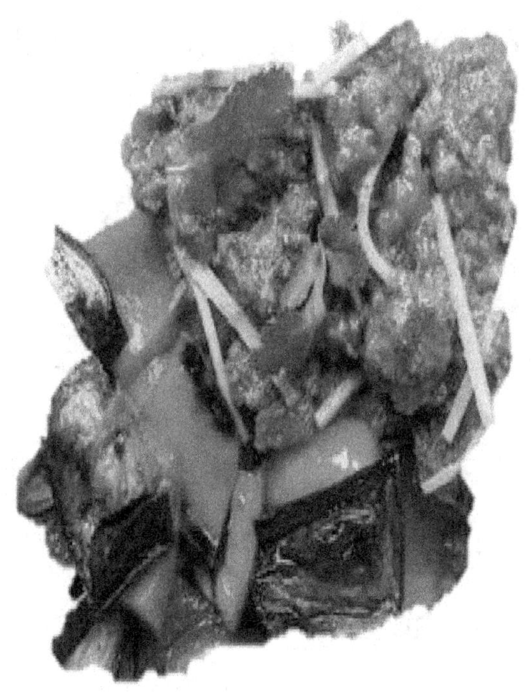

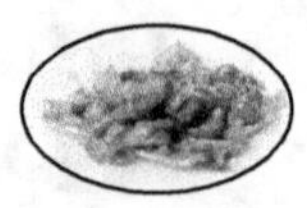 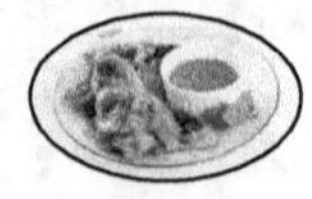 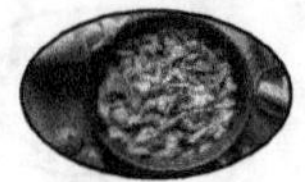

CONCLUSION

Irritable bowel syndrome and digestive issues can be effectively managed with the Low FODMAP Diet. Though challenging, the transition is possible with proper support. This book comprehensively covers the Low FODMAP Diet, providing advice on getting started, useful links, and recipes to simplify the process. Following this diet can bring relief and improve overall health with the right information and commitment.

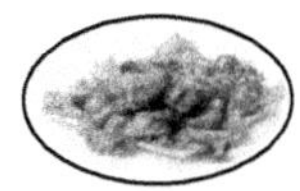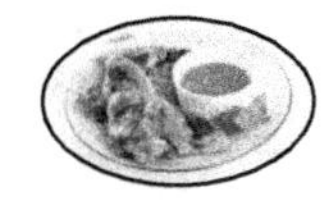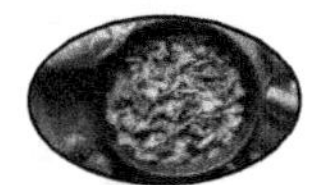

WE KNOW...

THAT'S WHY WE ARE SAYING THANK YOU...

"We know time is the unit of destiny, that's why we are saying thank you."

Dear Valued Customer,

we understand that time is a precious commodity, and we sincerely appreciate you choosing to spend a portion of it with us. Your decision to trust us with your purchase means the world to us, and we want to express our deepest gratitude.

Your support not only fuels our passion for delivering quality products but also contributes to the destiny of our business. Each customer is a vital part of our journey, and we are honored to have you

We strive to provide an exceptional shopping experience, and your satisfaction is our top priority. If you have any feedback or suggestions, we would love to hear from you. Your insights help us improve.

As a small token of our appreciation, we kindly invite you to share your experience by leaving a 5-star review. Your feedback not only boosts our morale but also assists fellow shoppers in making informed decisions.

Once again, thank you for choosing to buy this book. We look forward to serving you again and being a part of your destiny in the world of quality and excellence.

Warm regards,

Dr. Grace Hester–

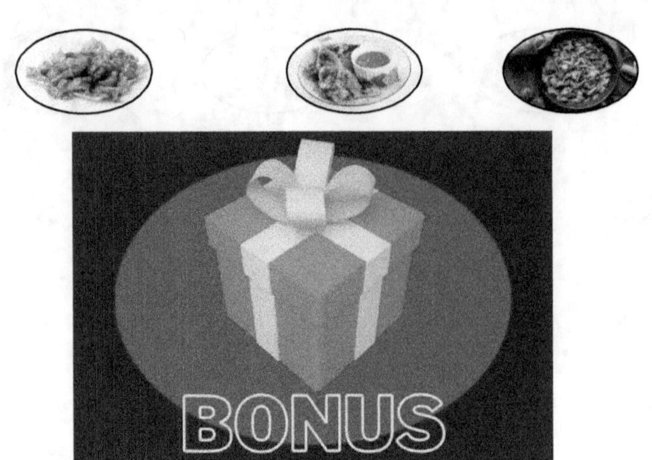

20 DAYS + MEAL PLANNER

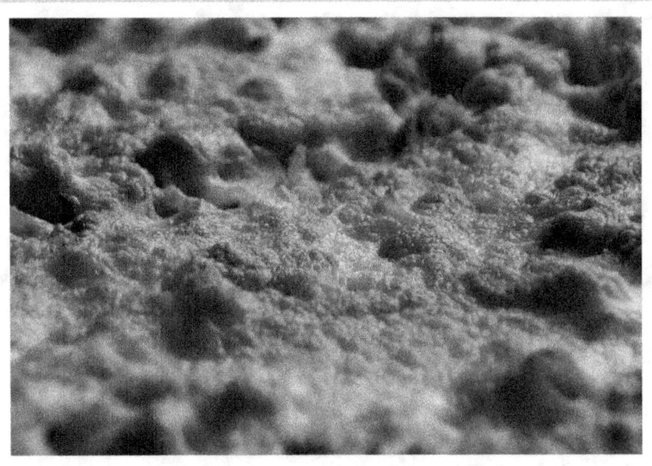

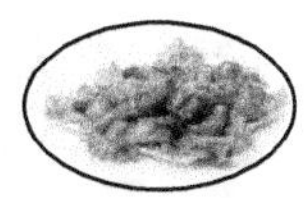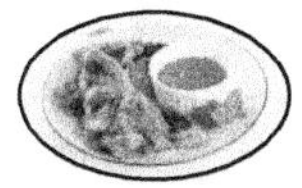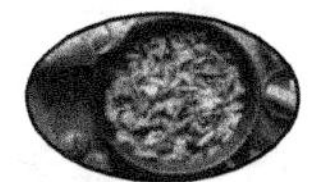

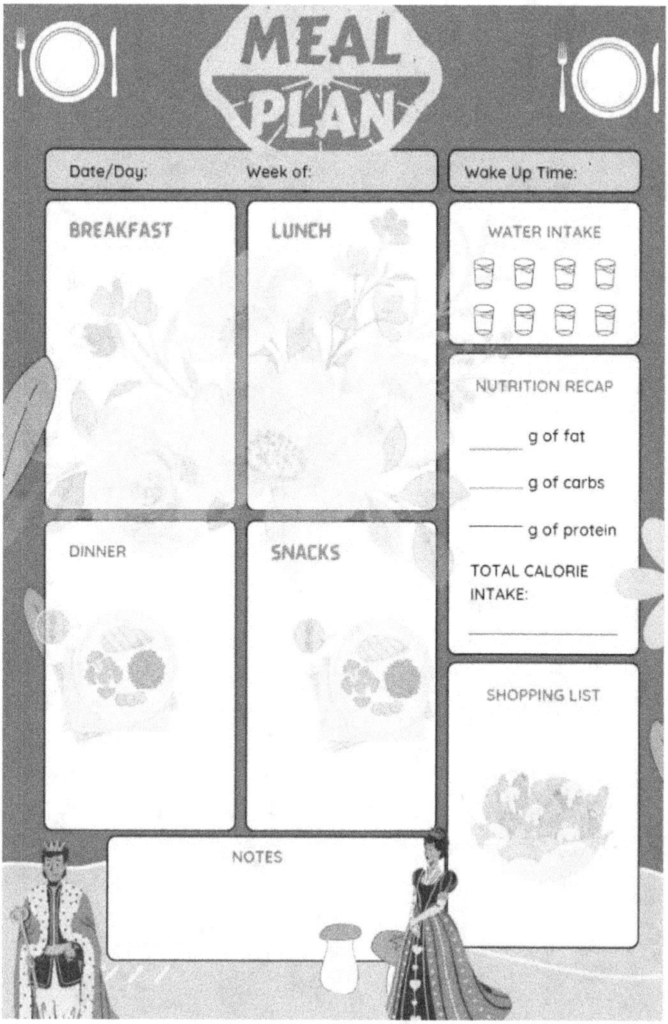

MEAL PLAN

| Date/Day: | Week of: | Wake Up Time: |

BREAKFAST

LUNCH

WATER INTAKE

NUTRITION RECAP

_______ g of fat

_______ g of carbs

_______ g of protein

TOTAL CALORIE INTAKE:

____

DINNER

SNACKS

SHOPPING LIST

NOTES

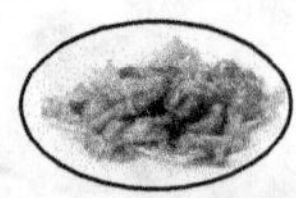
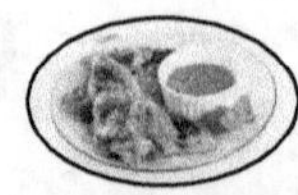
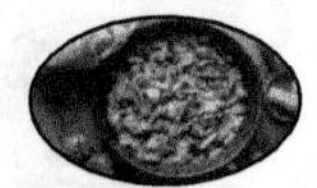

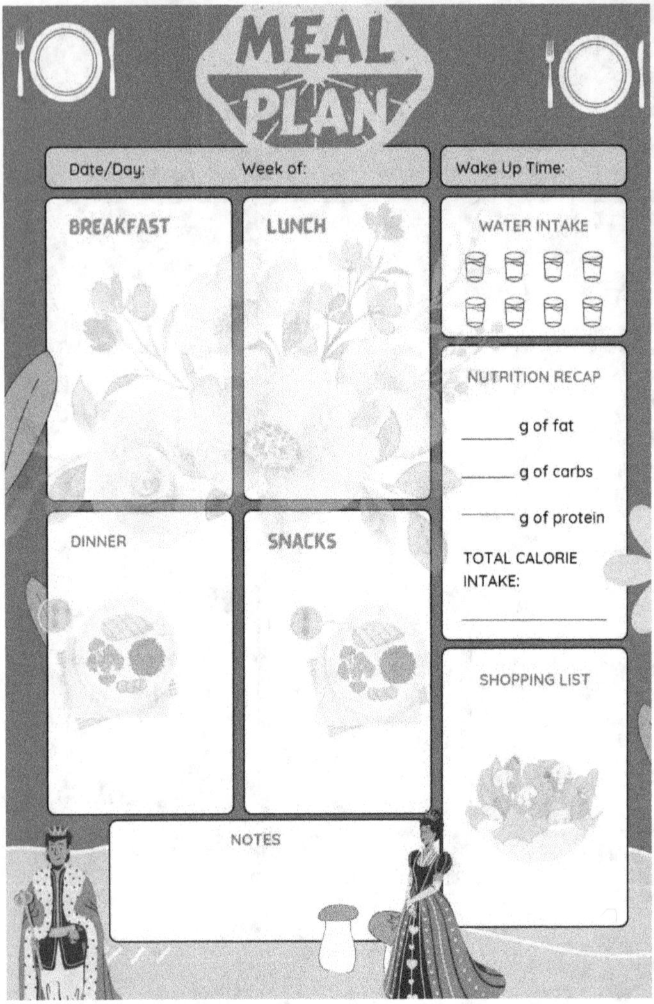

MEAL PLAN

| Date/Day: | Week of: | Wake Up Time: |

BREAKFAST

LUNCH

WATER INTAKE

NUTRITION RECAP

________ g of fat

________ g of carbs

________ g of protein

TOTAL CALORIE INTAKE:

____

DINNER

SNACKS

SHOPPING LIST

NOTES

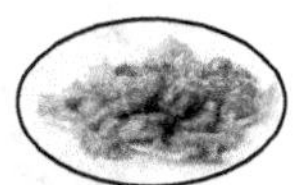 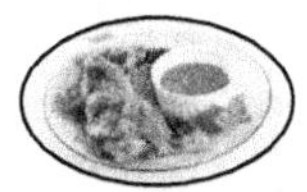 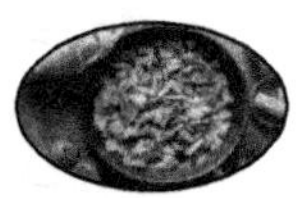

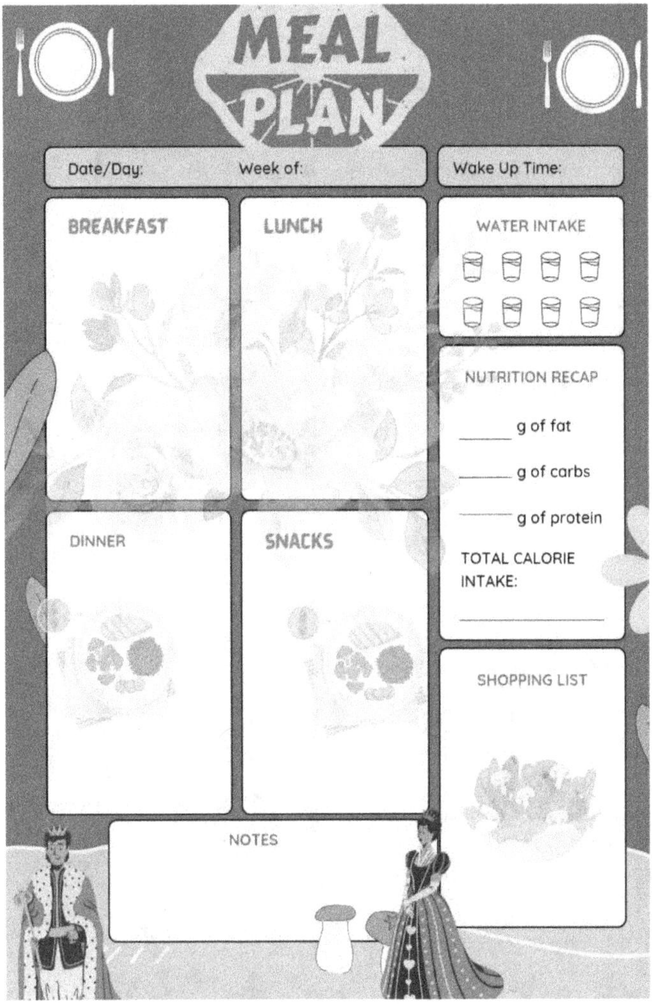

MEAL PLAN

Date/Day:	Week of:	Wake Up Time:

BREAKFAST

LUNCH

WATER INTAKE

NUTRITION RECAP

__________ g of fat

__________ g of carbs

__________ g of protein

TOTAL CALORIE INTAKE:

____

DINNER

SNACKS

SHOPPING LIST

NOTES

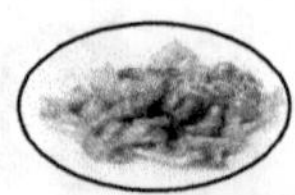 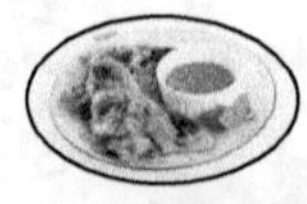 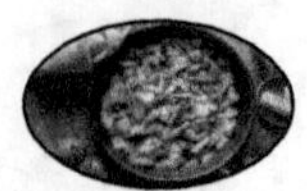

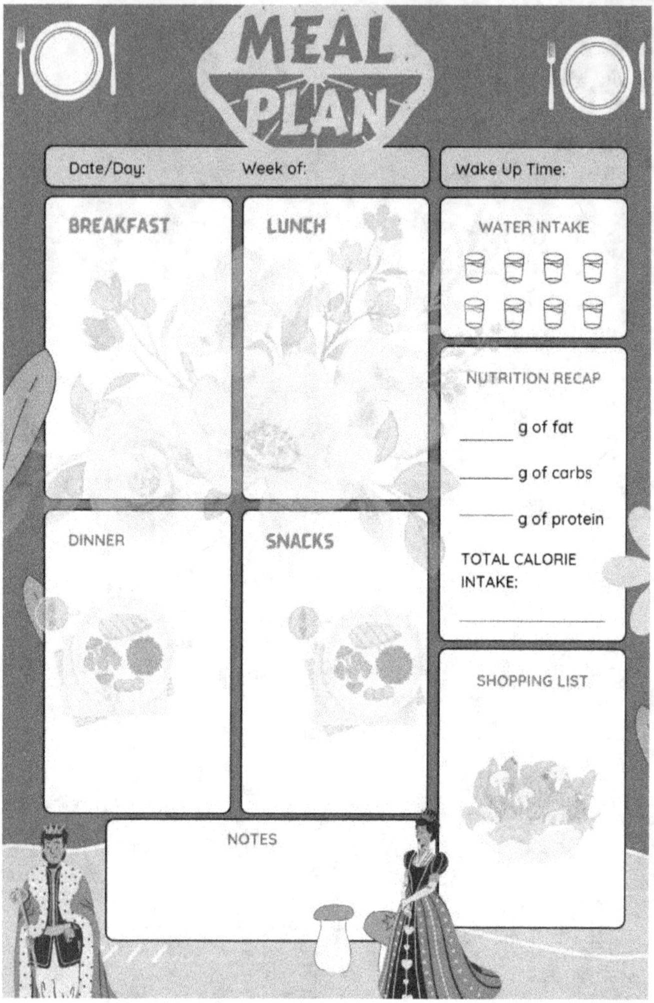

MEAL PLAN

Date/Day:	Week of:	Wake Up Time:

BREAKFAST

LUNCH

WATER INTAKE

NUTRITION RECAP

______ g of fat

______ g of carbs

______ g of protein

TOTAL CALORIE INTAKE:

____

DINNER

SNACKS

SHOPPING LIST

NOTES

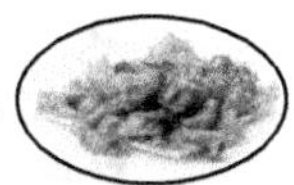 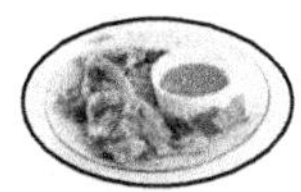 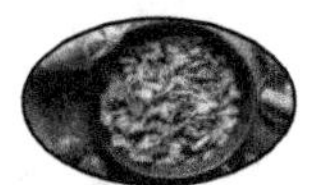

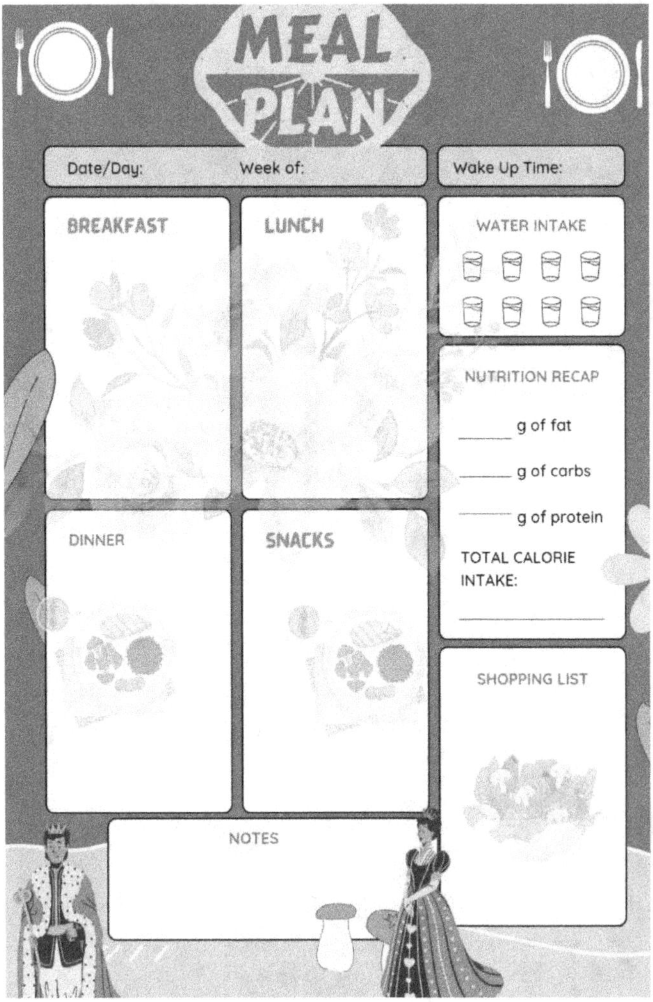

MEAL PLAN

| Date/Day: | Week of: | Wake Up Time: |

BREAKFAST

LUNCH

WATER INTAKE

NUTRITION RECAP

_______ g of fat

_______ g of carbs

_______ g of protein

TOTAL CALORIE INTAKE:

____

DINNER

SNACKS

SHOPPING LIST

NOTES

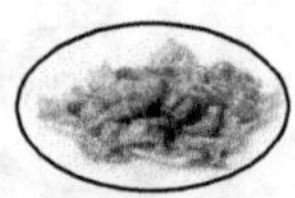
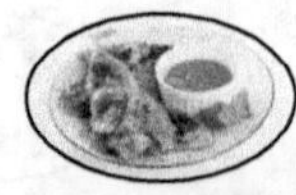
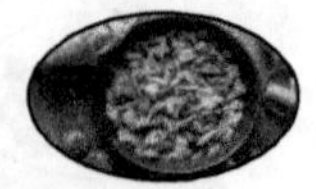

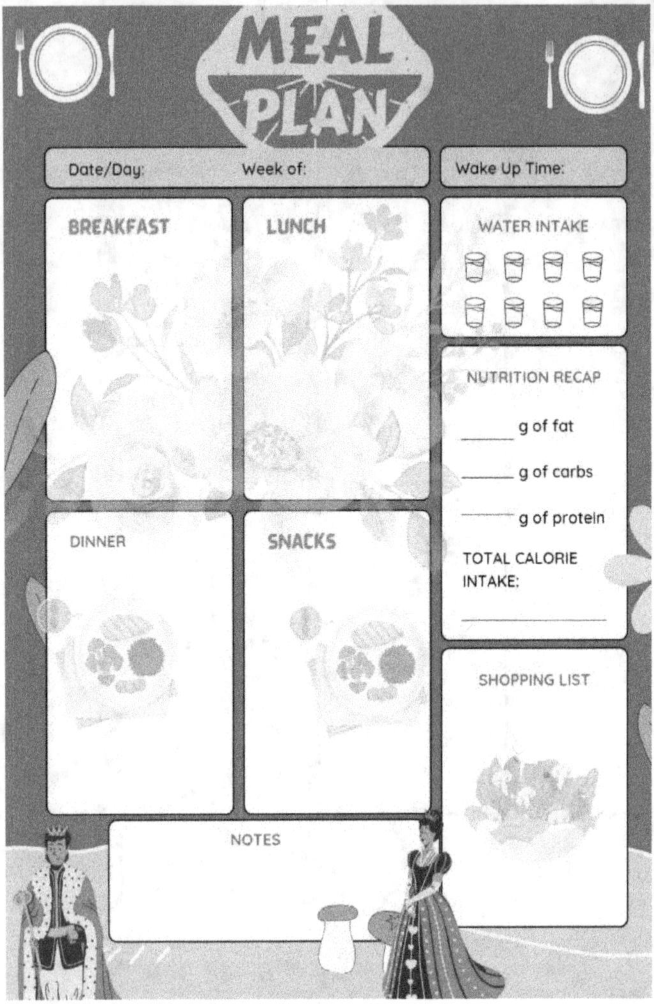

MEAL PLAN

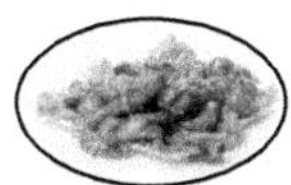 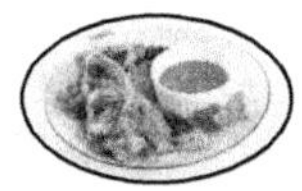 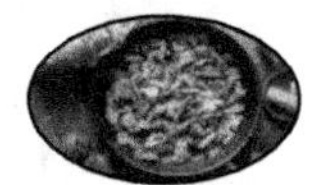

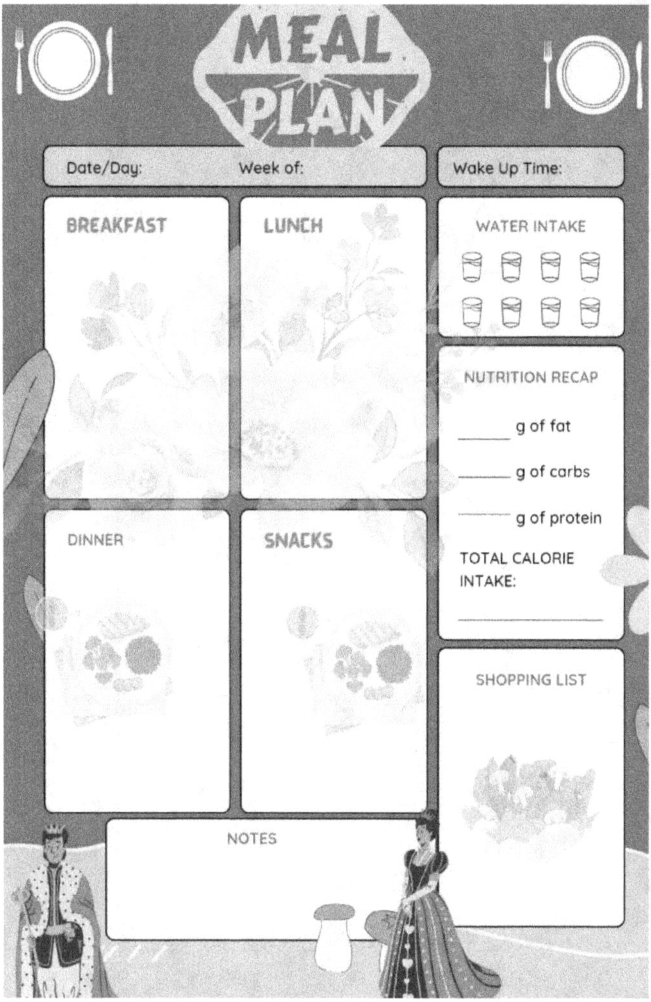

MEAL PLAN

Date/Day:	Week of:	Wake Up Time:

BREAKFAST

LUNCH

WATER INTAKE

NUTRITION RECAP

_______ g of fat

_______ g of carbs

_______ g of protein

TOTAL CALORIE INTAKE:

____

DINNER

SNACKS

SHOPPING LIST

NOTES

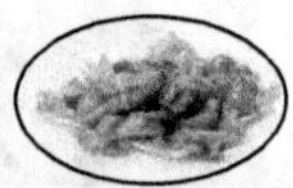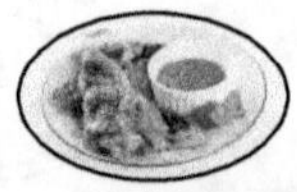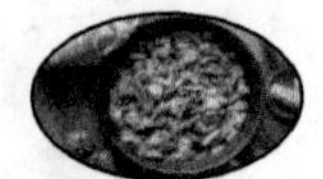

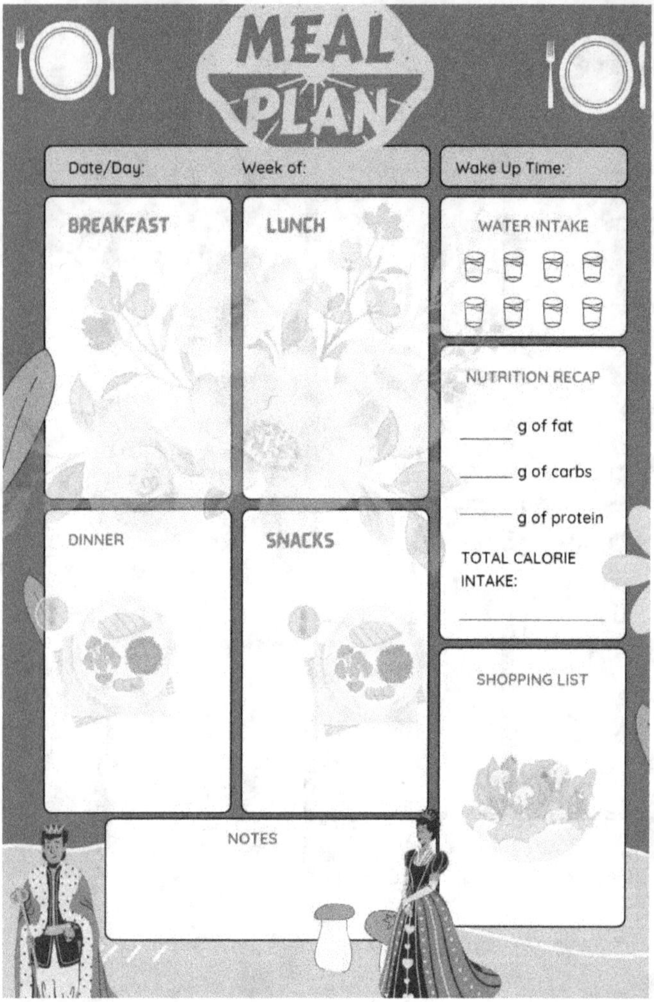

MEAL PLAN

| Date/Day: | Week of: | Wake Up Time: |

BREAKFAST

LUNCH

WATER INTAKE

NUTRITION RECAP

_______ g of fat

_______ g of carbs

_______ g of protein

TOTAL CALORIE INTAKE:

____

DINNER

SNACKS

SHOPPING LIST

NOTES

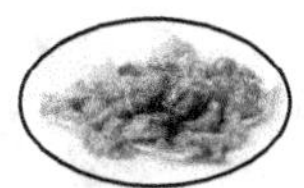
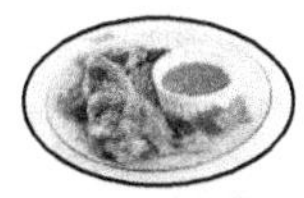
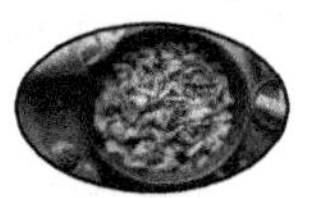

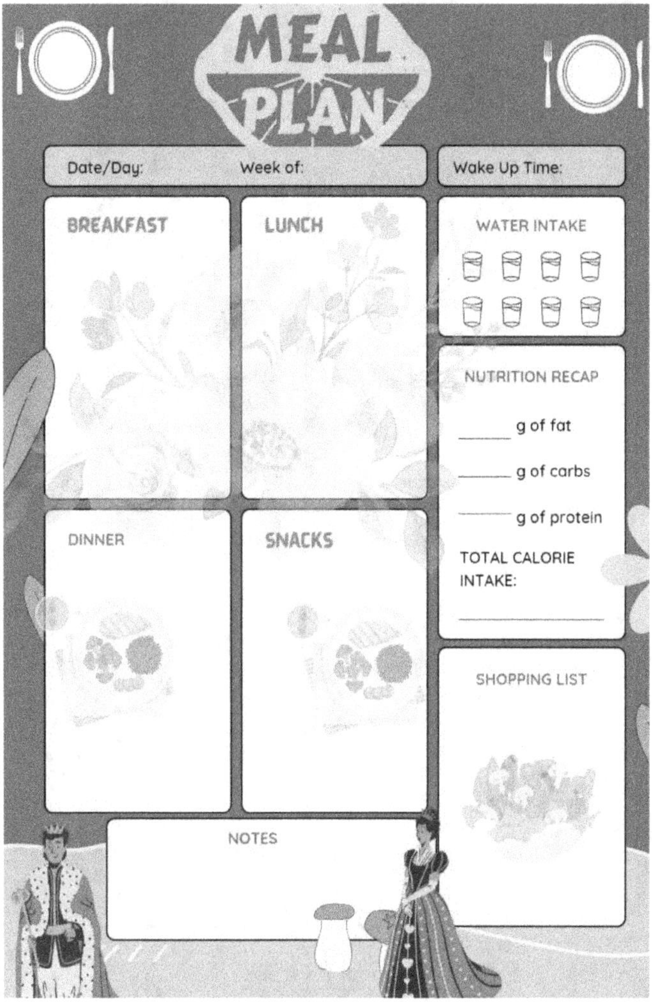

MEAL PLAN

Date/Day: Week of:

Wake Up Time:

BREAKFAST

LUNCH

WATER INTAKE

NUTRITION RECAP

_______ g of fat

_______ g of carbs

_______ g of protein

TOTAL CALORIE INTAKE:

____

DINNER

SNACKS

SHOPPING LIST

NOTES

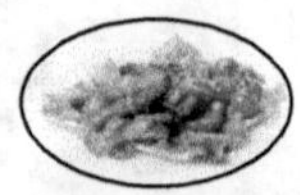 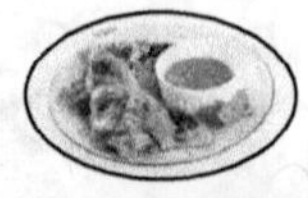 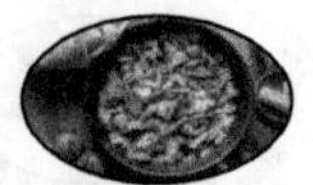

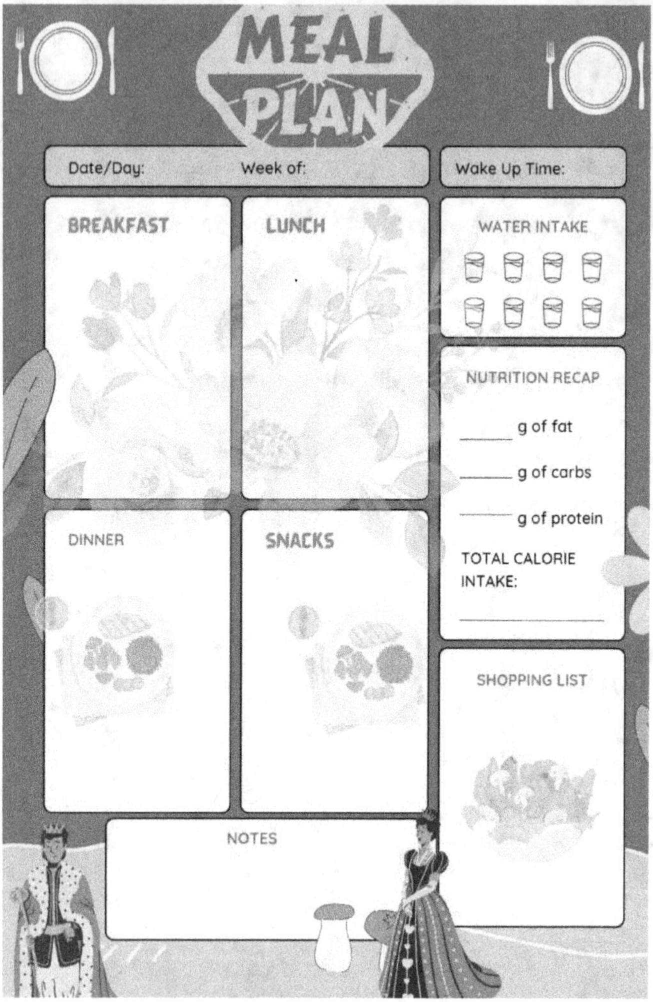

MEAL PLAN

Date/Day:	Week of:	Wake Up Time:

BREAKFAST

LUNCH

WATER INTAKE

NUTRITION RECAP

_______ g of fat

_______ g of carbs

_______ g of protein

TOTAL CALORIE INTAKE:

____

DINNER

SNACKS

SHOPPING LIST

NOTES

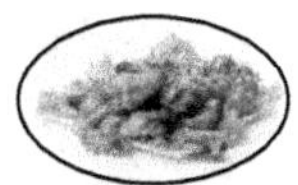
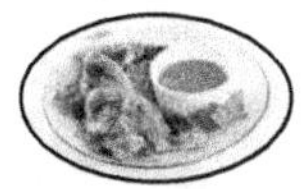
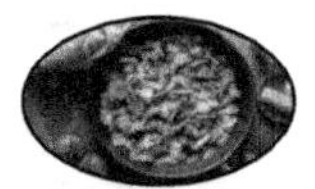

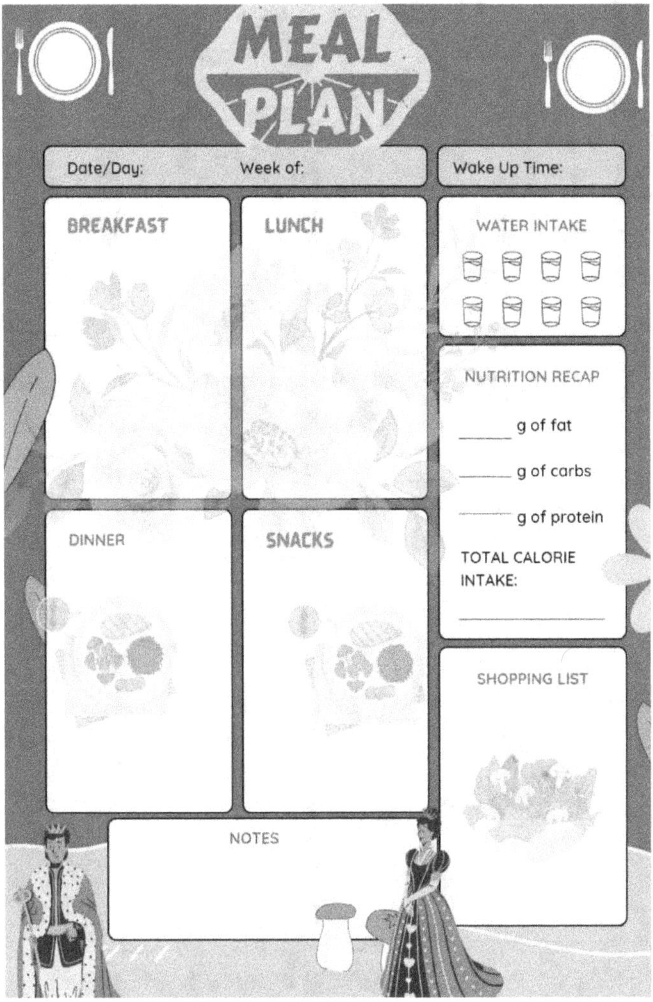

MEAL PLAN

| Date/Day: | Week of: | Wake Up Time: |

BREAKFAST

LUNCH

WATER INTAKE

NUTRITION RECAP

_______ g of fat

_______ g of carbs

_______ g of protein

TOTAL CALORIE INTAKE:

____

DINNER

SNACKS

SHOPPING LIST

NOTES

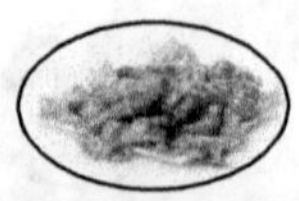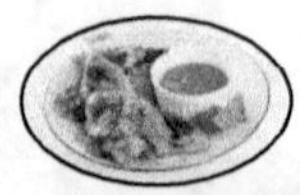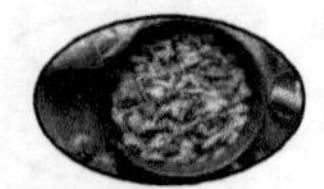

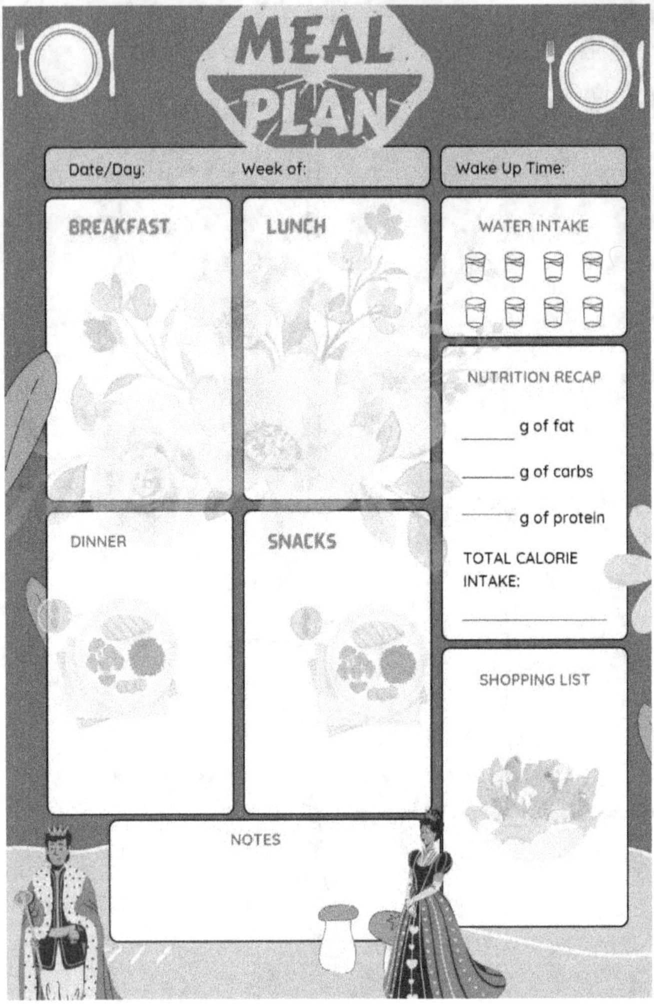

MEAL PLAN

Date/Day: Week of: Wake Up Time:

BREAKFAST

LUNCH

WATER INTAKE

NUTRITION RECAP

_______ g of fat

_______ g of carbs

_______ g of protein

TOTAL CALORIE INTAKE:

____

DINNER

SNACKS

SHOPPING LIST

NOTES

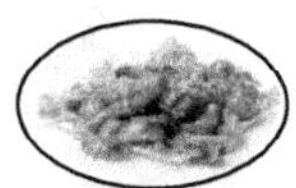 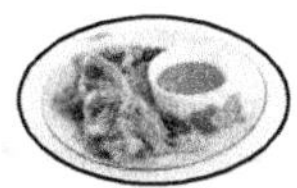 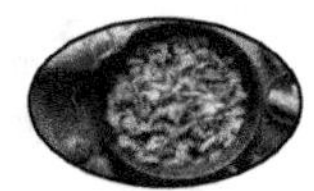

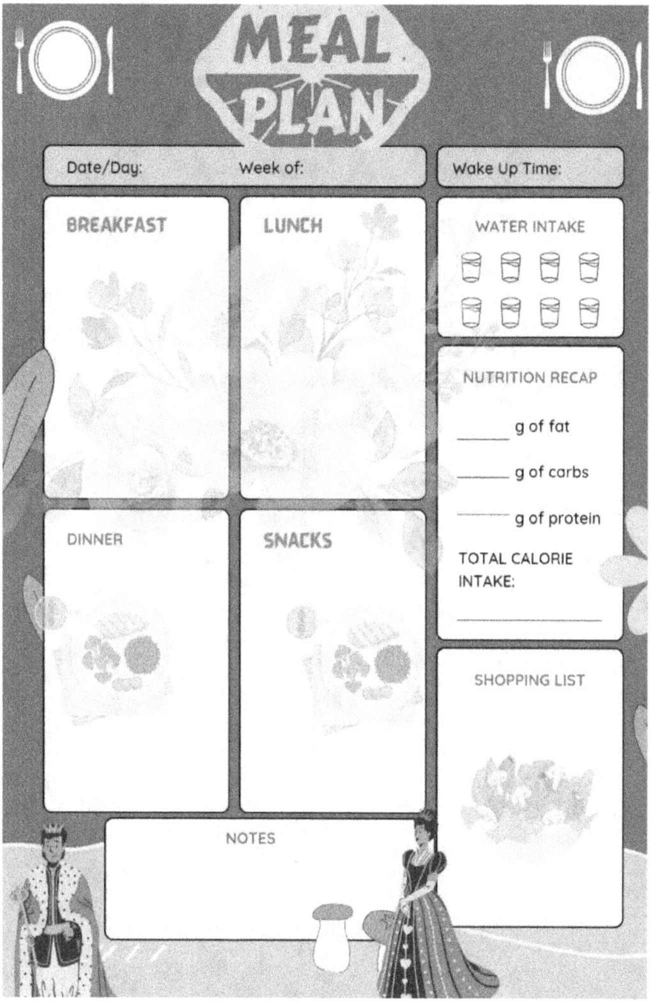

MEAL PLAN

Date/Day:	Week of:	Wake Up Time:

BREAKFAST

LUNCH

WATER INTAKE

NUTRITION RECAP

_________ g of fat

_________ g of carbs

_________ g of protein

TOTAL CALORIE INTAKE:

____

DINNER

SNACKS

SHOPPING LIST

NOTES

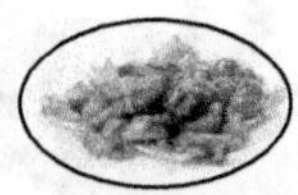 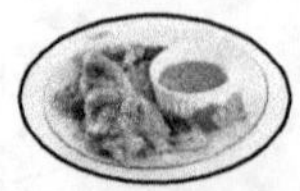 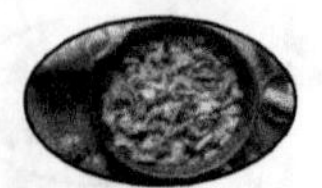

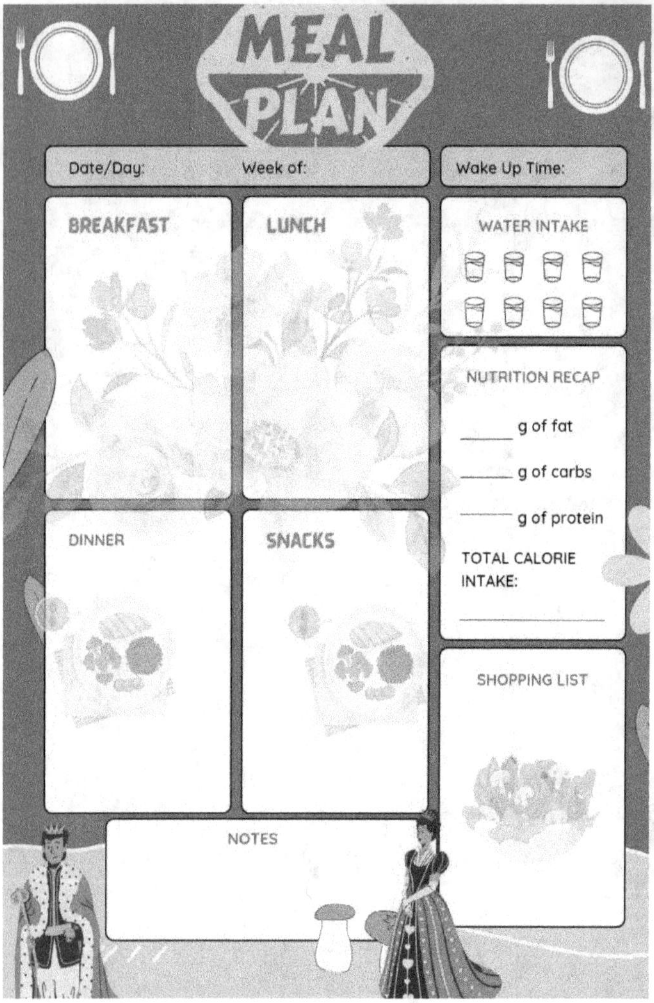

MEAL PLAN

Date/Day: Week of: Wake Up Time:

BREAKFAST

LUNCH

WATER INTAKE

NUTRITION RECAP

________ g of fat

________ g of carbs

________ g of protein

TOTAL CALORIE INTAKE:

____

DINNER

SNACKS

SHOPPING LIST

NOTES

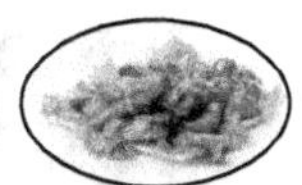 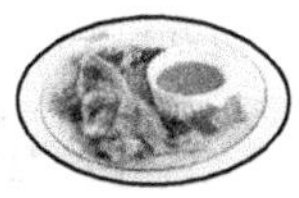 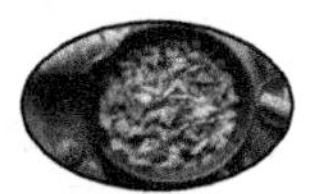

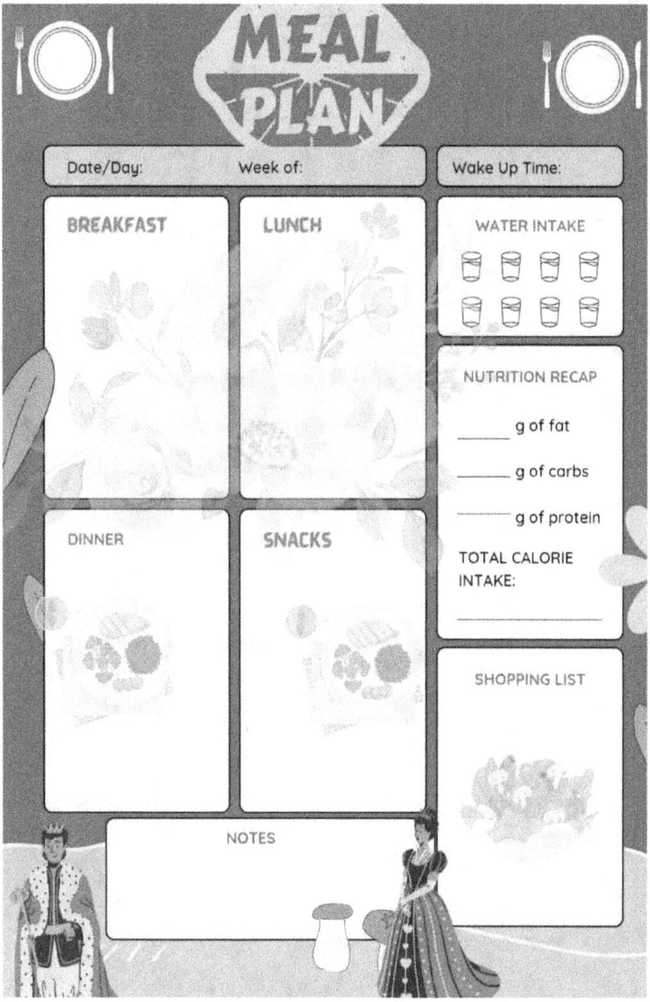

MEAL PLAN

Date/Day:	Week of:	Wake Up Time:

BREAKFAST

LUNCH

WATER INTAKE

NUTRITION RECAP

________ g of fat

________ g of carbs

________ g of protein

TOTAL CALORIE INTAKE:

____

DINNER

SNACKS

SHOPPING LIST

NOTES

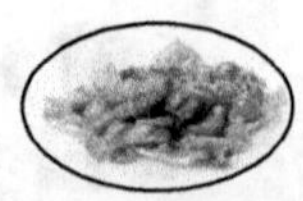 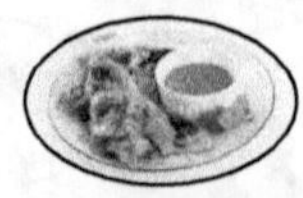 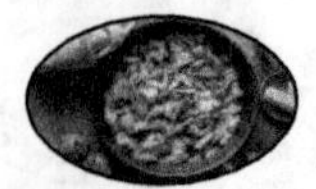

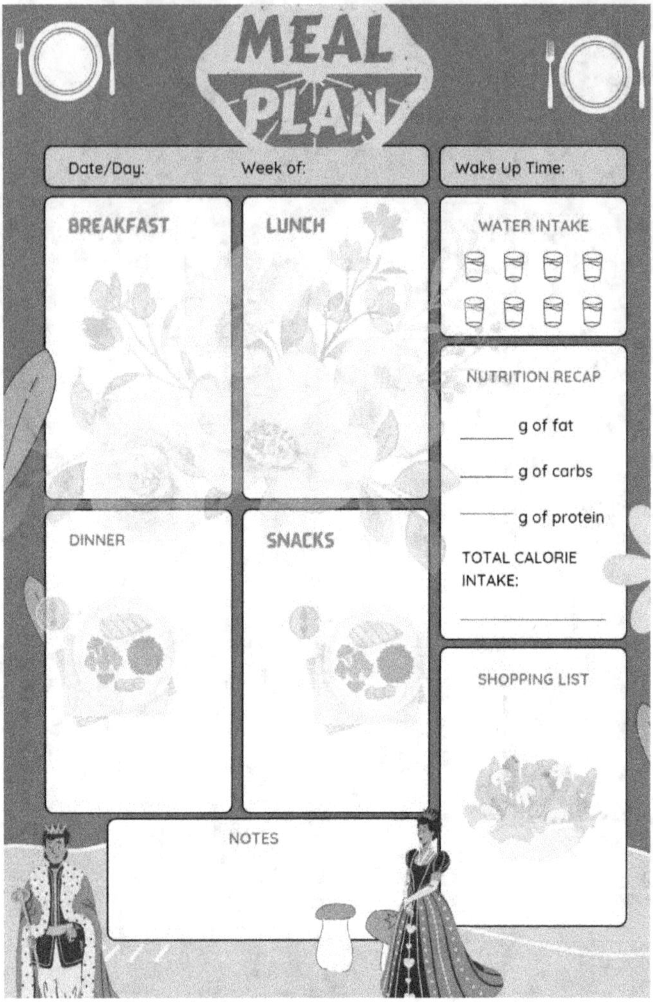

MEAL PLAN

| Date/Day: | Week of: | Wake Up Time: |

BREAKFAST

LUNCH

WATER INTAKE

NUTRITION RECAP

__________ g of fat

__________ g of carbs

__________ g of protein

TOTAL CALORIE INTAKE:

____

DINNER

SNACKS

SHOPPING LIST

NOTES

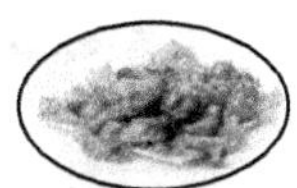
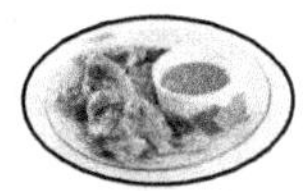
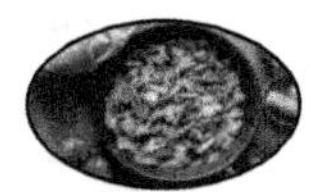

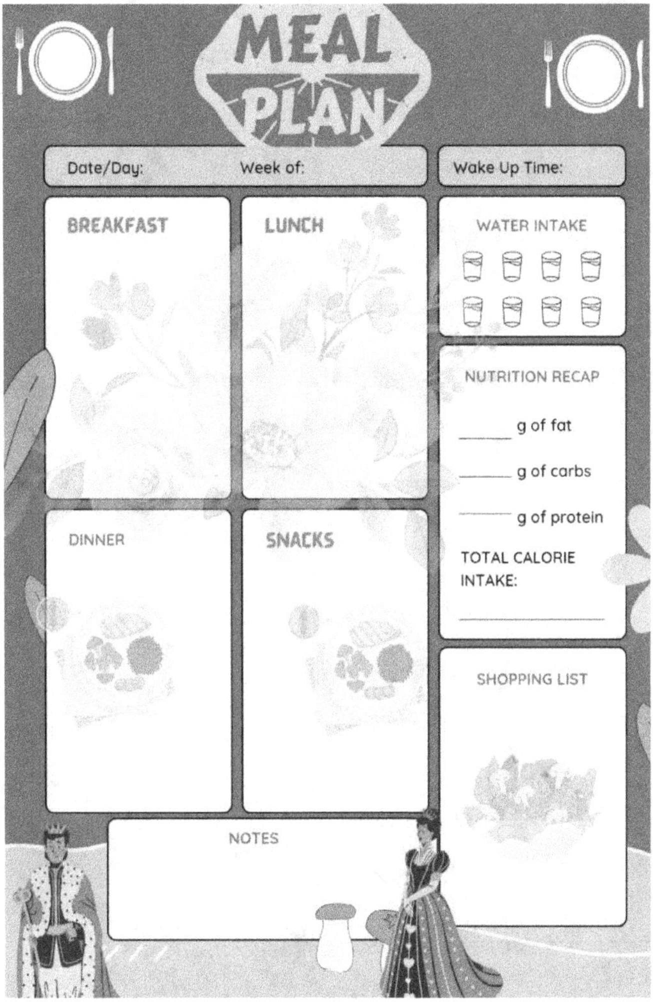

MEAL PLAN

Date/Day:	Week of:	Wake Up Time:

BREAKFAST

LUNCH

WATER INTAKE

NUTRITION RECAP

_______ g of fat

_______ g of carbs

_______ g of protein

TOTAL CALORIE INTAKE:

____

DINNER

SNACKS

SHOPPING LIST

NOTES

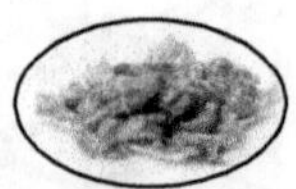 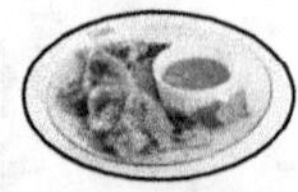 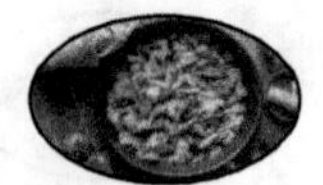

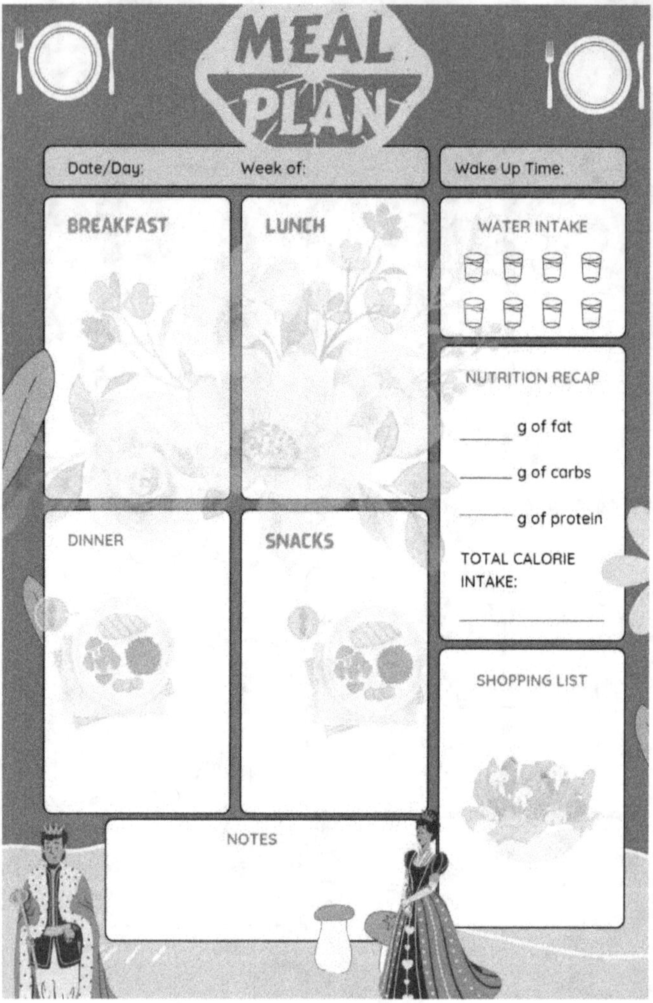

MEAL PLAN

| Date/Day: | Week of: | Wake Up Time: |

BREAKFAST

LUNCH

WATER INTAKE

NUTRITION RECAP

__________ g of fat

__________ g of carbs

__________ g of protein

TOTAL CALORIE INTAKE:

____

DINNER

SNACKS

SHOPPING LIST

NOTES

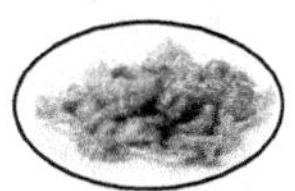
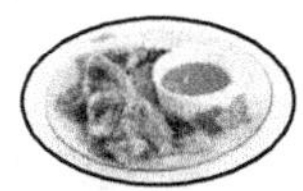
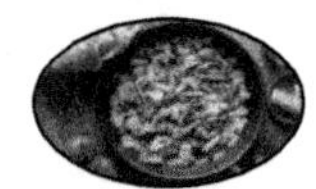

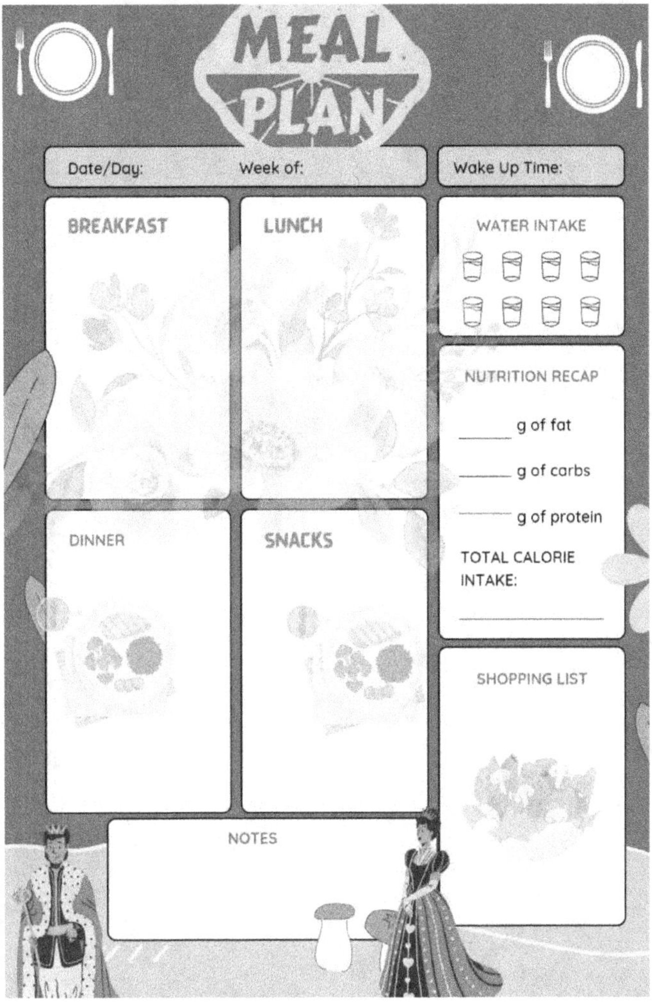

MEAL PLAN

| Date/Day: | Week of: | Wake Up Time: |

BREAKFAST

LUNCH

WATER INTAKE

NUTRITION RECAP

_______ g of fat

_______ g of carbs

_______ g of protein

TOTAL CALORIE INTAKE:

____

DINNER

SNACKS

SHOPPING LIST

NOTES